AIDS

The Politics and Policy of Disease

Stella Z. Theodoulou

California State University, Northridge

PRENTICE HALL, *Upper Saddle River, New Jersey 07458*

Library of Congress Cataloging-in-Publication Data

AIDS : the politics and policy of disease / Stella Z. Theodoulou.
    p. cm.
    Includes bibliographical references.
    ISBN 0–13–368630–2
    1. AIDS (Disease)— Government policy. 2. AIDS (Disease)—Social
aspects.   I. Theodoulou, Stella Z.
    RA644.A25A377   1996
    362.1'969792—dc20
                                           95–24865
                                                CIP

Acquisitions editor: Michael Bickerstaff
Editorial assistant: Anita Castro
Editoral/production supervision: Joseph Barron
Interior design: Peggy Gordon
Copy editor: William Stavru
Cover design: Bruce Kenselaar
Buyer: Bob Anderson

© 1996 by Prentice-Hall, Inc.
Simon & Schuster /A Viacom Company
Upper Saddle River, New Jersey 07458

Printed in the United States of America
10 9 8 7 6 5 4 3 2 1

ISBN 0-13-368630-2

Prentice-Hall International (UK) Limited, *London*
Prentice-Hall of Australia Pty. Limited, *Sydney*
Prentice-Hall Canada Inc., *Toronto*
Prentice-Hall Hispanoamericana, S.A., *Mexico*
Prentice-Hall of India Private Limited, *New Delhi*
Prentice-Hall of Japan, Inc., *Tokyo*
Simon & Schuster Asia Pte. Ltd., *Singapore*
Editora Prentice-Hall do Brasil, Ltda., *Rio de Janeiro*

To Dan and Guy, I miss you both; there are not enough words to describe your absence from this earth or my life.

This book is dedicated to both of you and to everyone fighting for their lives against this virus.

Contents

Preface

The AIDS epidemic offers political scientists the opportunity to ask a variety of questions about politics and policy and to do so from every subfield of the discipline. The political ramifications of AIDS are a daily media item, and like many other topics covered in political science courses, AIDS has an immediate and direct bearing on the lives of all of us. The ramifications of the disease will accompany each of us throughout the next decades. Thus, it is vital that the AIDS crisis be examined within the context of the political science curriculum and that there be material that addresses the subject from a purely political perspective. The purpose of this reader is to help students understand the political and policy dimensions of the epidemic.

The reader emerges from a course that I have developed and taught at California State University, Northridge, and reflects key contemporary research on the epidemic from a broad variety of policy and political perspectives. At the same time, it shares a common understanding of AIDS as a fundamentally challenging issue that calls for a highly political response.

The readings are grouped into three broad sections. Part One covers the political dimension of AIDS. Readings deal with ethical considerations, constitutional issues, the bureaucratic dimension, the contradictions in delivery of public health services in a capitalist economy, the position of the disease within the current institutional and economic crisis of nonprosperous America, and the actors involved in the AIDS issue arena. The second part of the reader deals with the policy dimension of AIDS. Readings focus on the nature and dynamics of the policy process in relation to the disease, and on the evaluation of various governmental responses with respect to the criteria of effectiveness, justice, equity and ethical acceptability based on the principles of respect for the individual, harm, beneficence, and fairness. Part Three deals with the comparative dimension of AIDS and looks at how other nations have responded to the demands of the epidemic.

Finally, I would like to express my thanks and appreciation to the following individuals. To my research assistant, Gloria Guevara: this text would not have been possible without your insights and hard work. To Amanda Potter and my cousin Stella Theodoulou, both of London Guildhall University: your editorial comments were invaluable. To my editors and Prentice Hall representative Marcy Pearlman: your determination to see this in print was tenacious. To my reviewers, Patricia Freeman of the University of Tennessee, John Whitney of Lincoln Land Community College, and George Frederickson of the University of Kansas: thank you for your time and consideration. To CSUN colleagues Gene Price and Matt Cahn: your presence and friendship are appreciated. And finally, but not least, to Marti: nothing is possible without you.

Stella Z. Theodoulou

PART ONE

The Politics of AIDS

1

AIDS Equals Politics

Stella Z. Theodoulou

AIDS the disease is unconcerned with politics, social status, or sexual preference. AIDS the national health crisis illuminates some troubling biases and discriminatory practices in the American economic, political, social, and health care systems (Cropley, 1991; Gostin, 1989; Patton, 1990). The politics of the disease raise a number of complex ethical, political, and policy issues. Thus, to understand the policy stream surrounding acquired immune deficiency syndrome (AIDS) one has to comprehend that the disease is not merely a health care issue, it also involves the issues of racism, sexism, sexual preference, and classism (Altman, 1986; Somerville & Orkin, 1989; Stuntzner-Gibson, 1991). AIDS and its implications for a mass society span every cleavage in American society. What is unique, terrifying, and challenging about the epidemic is its position within the prevailing institutional and economic crisis of nonprosperous America. The disarray caused by the disease in the last decade can be seen mainly in America's unfulfilled housing, education, and physical and mental health care needs. AIDS should be viewed as a primary failure of the human immune system and of the polity.

This epidemic offers political scientists the opportunity to ask a variety of questions about politics and power. Thus, this study looks at AIDS as a political and policy phenomenon rather then as a health issue. Within such an analysis attention is paid to the contradictions in the delivery of public health services in a capitalist economy. This study is concerned with the policy response of the American federal government and as such, does not attempt to look at any AIDS related laws or local policy arrangements that have been formulated and implemented.

AIDS: A PANDEMIC RUNNING WILD

AIDS is a medical condition caused by the human immunodeficiency virus (HIV; Buehler, 1990; Duesberg, 1989; Fauci, 1988; Safyer & Spies-Karotkin, 1988); however, there has been increasing debate about whether HIV does in fact cause AIDS. The global AIDS epidemic is volatile, dynamic, and unstable, and its major impacts are yet to come. As of January 1994, 22.2 million people around the world (8.7 million women, 11.3 million men, and 2.2 million children) have been infected with HIV. Of approximately 35% of these people in whom AIDS has developed, more than 70% have died (Centers for Disease Control and Prevention, 1994). Table 1–1 shows the distribution of the cumulative number of HIV–infected people for ten geographical areas.

When one looks at the future the numbers become increasingly uncertain due to differences in forecasting techniques. According to the most conservative forecasts, by the year 2000 a minimum of 38 million adults will have become HIV–positive. A more liberal forecast puts the figure as high as 110 million (Mann et al., 1992).

In the United States, as of September 1994, approximately 424,000 individuals have contracted AIDS; of these, nearly 77% are now dead (Kirp & Bayer, 1992; Gladwell, 1993; Herek & Capitanio, 1993). Data show that perhaps as many as 3 to 6 million Americans are infected by the HIV virus (Centers for Disease Control and Prevention, 1994).

The numbers both globally and in America are indeed intimidating and from them the basic traits of the AIDS pandemic can be discerned. No nation in the world can claim that it has stopped the spread of HIV and AIDS. The virus is spreading globally; AIDS cases have been officially reported by 164 nations, and HIV infection has been documented in practically all nations (Mann et al., 1992). As the epidemic evolves it also becomes more complicated with time. From this, many have concluded that the AIDS pandemic is now out of control (Mann et al., 1992; Kirp & Bayer, 1992; Palca, 1991). Indeed, on January 27, 1994, at an AIDS fund raiser in Los Angeles, former AIDS Coordinator, Kristine Gebbie announced, "We do have a long way to go here. It took us 12 years to acknowledge it's an epidemic, now it's just out of control."

THE DEMOGRAPHICS OF HIV/AIDS

AIDS does not discriminate on the basis of race, gender, class, geography, or sexuality. In spite of the myth that has been perpetuated by many of the so-called "moral majority," AIDS is not a "gay plague" (Grutsch & Robertson,

TABLE 1-1 Cumulative HIV Infection in Adults & Children by Geographical Area of Affinity (GAA), 1994 & 1996 (projected)

	Men		Women		Children		Total	
	1994	1996 (projected)	1994	1996 (projected)	1994	1996 (projected)	1994	1996 (projected)
North America	963,000	1,087,000	160,000	181,000	14,000	18,000	1,138,000	1,286,000
Western Europe	545,000	691,000	109,000	138,000	6,000	9,000	660,000	838,000
Oceania	24,000	28,000	3,000	3,000	<1,000	<1,000	27,000	32,000
Latin America	1,002,000	1,182,000	250,000	295,000	61,000	79,000	1,313,000	1,556,000
Sub-Saharan Africa	6,411,000	7,881,000	7,052,000	8,670,000	1,996,000	2,672,000	15,459,000	19,222,000
Caribbean	225,000	280,000	150,000	187,000	26,000	36,000	402,000	503,000
Eastern Europe	25,000	30,000	3,000	3,000	<1,000	<1,000	28,000	34,000
SE Mediterranean	47,000	59,000	9,000	12,000	2,000	2,000	58,000	73,000
Northeast Asia	77,000	149,000	15,000	30,000	1,000	2,000	94,000	181,000
Southeast Asia	1,968,000	6,236,000	984,000	3,118,000	68,000	251,000	3,020,000	9,605,000
Total World	11,287,000	17,623,000	8,737,000	12,637,000	2,175,000	3,070,000	22,200,000	33,330,000

Source: Data from Global AIDS Policy Coalition, *AIDs in the World*, Vol. II (Oxford: Oxford University Press, 1995).

1986). In Africa and Asia the majority of people with HIV and AIDS are heterosexual (Table 1–2).

Current data show that in the United States the virus affects African Americans and Hispanics at higher rates than Caucasians. It is growing rapidly among women in the 18 to 35 age bracket. One in 5 people with AIDS are between the ages of 20 to 29 (Centers for Disease Control and Prevention, 1994; Ehrhardt, 1992; Maticka-Tyndale, 1992). Homosexual and bisexual men are still the group, within the United States, with the highest incidence of infection, although changes in behavior within the homosexual population have resulted in lower incidences of new infections than in most other demographic groups. 1993/1994 witnessed a one percent decrease in the rate of growth of homosexual and bisexual transmission. The total number of such cases in 1993 was 30,300 (CDC, 1994). Indeed, the largest increase in new cases of infection have been in the general heterosexual population. In 1993/1994 heterosexual transmission of AIDS cases in the United States grew by 23 percent to 7,500 cases (CDC, 1994).

When all things are held equal, the most important identifying variable is income. Regardless of race, orientation, or language, those in the lower socioeconomic brackets are more likely to have HIV (Freudenberg, 1990; Huber & Schnerder, 1992; Strauss, 1991). As the epidemic spreads, it is becoming more and more a disease that can affect any American regardless of sexual preference or race, but in particular it is becoming more and more a disease of the poor, the group within American society that has inadequate access to health care (Smith, 1993). And where HIV is becoming more a disease of heterosexuals, it is becoming also more a disease of women, because

TABLE 1–2 Percentage of HIV–Infected Individuals by Mode of Transmission in Adults by Geographic Area of Affinity (GAA), 1992

GAA	Mode of Transmission %	
	Heterosexual	Homosexual
North America	9	56
Western Europe	14	47
Oceania	6	87
Latin America	24	54
Sub-Saharan Africa	93	1
Caribbean	75	10
Eastern Europe	10	80
Southeastern Mediterranean	20	35
North East Asia	50	20
South East Asia	70	8

Source: Data from Mann et al. (eds.), 1992.

transmission to women from heterosexual contact is easier than for men (Novello, 1991; Shayne, 1991). One must also remember that women are disproportionately represented among those living in poverty in the United States. As the epidemic increases globally, it is becoming more and more a disease of the third world (Desvarieux & Pape, 1991).

The impact of the epidemic is unique. Unlike malaria or polio—previous modern epidemics—, it principally affects young and middle-aged adults. This is not only the sexually most active years for individuals, but also their prime productive and reproductive years. Thus, the impact of AIDS is demographic, economic, and social. AIDS is a disease of human groups and its demographic and social impacts multiply from the infected individual to the group. In the most affected areas infant, child, and adult mortality is rising, and life expectancy at birth is declining rapidly (Mann et al., 1992). The cost of medical care for each patient overwhelms individuals and households. And everywhere the response of governments is cut from the same cloth.

THE GOVERNMENTAL RESPONSE TO AIDS

Every nation has had to devise policies suited to its own political, economic, and cultural conditions. Kirp and Bayer (1992) argue that a wide spectrum of AIDS policies can be found in the industrialized democracies; however, what all nations share in common is the epidemic's position as a part of the domestic political agenda and a center of ideological conflict.

The United States' response to the epidemic has, like other industrialized democracies, been affected by cultural factors. AIDS is much more than a challenge to medical science, it is linked to the controversial subjects of sex and drugs, and because the disease surfaced first among homosexual Americans and drug users, it provoked deep and complicated feelings in everyone that have extended across our society with political and social consequences and deep ramifications. Basically, AIDS has tested the nation's abilities to act responsibly and sanely in the face of catastrophe.

What has occurred in the United States is a division of labor between the government and the private and voluntary sectors. The political response has been one of bewilderment and inconsistency. Most of the achievements have come from the private sector. Although the federal government has finally acknowledged AIDS as an epidemic, there has been no overall national governmental strategy to overcome it. Many authors have characterized the American government's response as a failure of leadership (Freudenberg, 1990; Gostin, 1989; Kirp & Bayer, 1992; Shilts, 1987).

Many gay activists have argued that the response in the United States has been plagued by two themes. The first is apathy on the part of the federal government. At best, the government has been negligent; at worst, it has aggravated the epidemic. In many instances the government has stood in the way of forces and developments that many have argued might have proved beneficial (Epstein, 1991; Kramer, 1990; Shilts, 1987). There has been little planning, counseling, or coordination. Indeed, the American government for most of the first decade of the epidemic can be charged with irresponsibility.

The second theme is the growth of a grass roots, private, voluntary sector. In the long run such a sector is limited, but the growth and accomplishments of such organizations tell a lesson. Such a sector permits greater diversity and experimentation. Private organizations allow for more flexibility and rapid absorption of changes then government bureaucracies. They also give communities—such as homosexuals—more voice in shaping solutions to problems that face them in particular (Arno, 1986; Mcguire, 1989; Payne, 1992). The weakness of relying on the private sector's response to the epidemic is that this sector took responsibility for much of what the national government should have been doing policywise.

The response by government in the United States is not surprising during the early years of the epidemic. Most of the political attention upon AIDS came from conservative political groups and candidates seeking the electoral support of such voters. AIDS presented society with a disease that seemed to bear out everything that the New Right stood for and supported. The disease proved useful to the Right in three distinct ways. First, AIDS promoted the argument that the nation was suffering heavily from the excesses of the sexual revolution, the increased willingness to recognize and lend legitimacy to the "gay lifestyle," and greater tolerance of and participation in recreational drugs. Second, it permitted homosexuals and drug users to be represented and characterized as despicable, dirty, and virulent, an enemy within. Third, because of its salience in certain racial minorities, AIDS also surfaced in the context of race relations.

AIDS became a litmus test by which candidates for office were judged (Kirp & Bayer, 1992; Shilts, 1987; Wachter, 1992). If a candidate was not perceived as "tough" on AIDS, then he or she was clearly in favor of homosexuality, drug use, immorality, and decadence. In the first half of the 1980s, candidates of both parties took a hard line on AIDS and this meant the advocation of mandatory testing, the reporting of those infected, and the isolation of all individuals who were infected. Compounding this was sensational media coverage and a frenzy of misinformation or noninformation. The result was inevitable; no administration, let alone a conservative one, would act to formulate and implement a national policy. Also, in such a climate it is not surprising that a feeling of hate and overt "bashing" of homosexuals would develop. This climate is witnessed by an incredible rise in the number of hate crimes against gays (Crimp & Rolston, 1990).

Indicative of this anti–AIDS environment was Ronald Reagan's refusal to publicly acknowledge the disease or its epidemic level. In fact, it was not until 1987 that President Reagan spoke out publicly about the disease. This was some six years after the virus was first publicly acknowledged. One must ask why the change? The answer lies in a change within the environment of infection. By the late 1980s conservatives found it increasingly more difficult to obtain the sort of political capital from AIDS that they had in the first part of the decade, due to the lessening of the panic rhetoric that once marked the debate. America had not been overrun with victims of the disease—although the numbers of HIV–infected people and AIDs–related deaths were staggering—and AIDS was no longer a "purely" gay disease. Thanks to the emergence of Ryan White, a heterosexual teenager who had become infected through blood transfusion, and basketball hero Magic Johnson's announcement of his HIV infection from multiple heterosexual sexual relations, it was now perceived that AIDS was no longer confined to any specific segment of society (Kalichman, 1992). This realization forced America to look at AIDS in a different light. No longer could heterosexual America take comfort in the belief that this was a disease to which they were immune. It was now acceptable to suggest AIDS might be a public health problem that government should act upon. Hence, Reagan's appointment of a Presidential Commission to investigate and make policy recommendations on the epidemic.

By the start of the 1990s it was fashionable for politicians to openly support funding for AIDS research and AIDS antidiscrimination legislation. In 1990 Congress voted overwhelmingly in favor of an AIDS disaster bill that sought between 3 to 4 billion dollars to be spent on research, treatment, education, and prevention over a five-year period. At the same time, Congress also passed the Americans with Disabilities Act that aimed to protect the civil rights of all disabled citizens. There was general acknowledgment that this should include AIDS patients and HIV–infected individuals.

The politicization of AIDS was also largely due to the mobilization of the homosexual community. In the early years this community was largely committed to caring for their own rather than articulating that AIDS was a political problem. With the emergence of the militant group ACT UP the homosexual community mobilized behind a political platform. The platform became the basis of a new activist gay agenda. Among the demands were the following: no apology for homosexuality, the protection and advancement of civil rights, and political action to deal with the epidemic. The basis of the platform was the belief by gay activists, such as Larry Kramer, that it was only through political action that the system would respond to the needs of HIV and AIDS victims in a timely and meaningful fashion, and that only if gays were guaranteed the same civil rights as heterosexuals could this become a reality. Despite its notoriety, in both heterosexual and homosexual society, ACT UP has managed to achieve a number of important victories. For example, due to the mobilization of gays the Food and Drug Administration (FDA) was forced to speed up the approval of new drugs such as AZT. However, in the last year or so, this particular drug and its FDA approval have come under increasing criticism (Arno & Feiden, 1993).

At this point it would be useful to summarize the reasons for the failure of leadership and the absence of the formulation and implementation of a national AIDS policy. First, when the disease first hit, it most deeply affected groups outside mainstream America. As it progressed it then hit most heavily in racial minorities. Homosexuals, drug users, African Americans, and Hispanics have few political representatives and few advocates. Such groups and their "lifestyles" are viewed by many in "white middle America" with distaste and disapproval. The next reason for the failure of leadership is the inadequacy of the American health care system. It is a system in which primary health care medicine is in a crisis and unable to manage long-term and debilitating disease (Smith, 1993). On top of this, private health insurance has been swamped and is reluctant to provide, maintain, or honor coverage for those infected with the disease. Compounding these problems is the fact that those groups who tend to be uninsured or underinsured are also those groups who need adequate access to health care. (Aukerman, 1991; Davis & Rowland, 1991; Fain, 1993; Hurowitz, 1993; Manuel, 1991). These are the very same groups that the epidemic has hit the hardest.

AIDS has created a tremendous strain on the American public and private health care systems. Most of the problems have been dealt with on a temporary basis (Cockerell & Nary, 1991). AIDS needs long-term care, an added burden that many refuse to acknowledge. It should be clear to everyone that there is no simple answer to the health crisis that America faces. The obstacles to establishing effective public health policies are considerable as the Clinton administration would be the first to admit.

Unfortunately, AIDS is a disease with a unique set of public health problems. The United States has relatively little recent experience dealing with health crises. Since the introduction of antibiotics during the Second World War, health priorities shifted to chronic systemic diseases. Until the 1980s, infectious epidemic disease was seen as a thing of the past or a concern of the developing world. Thus, many have looked to the past for historical models as a means of dealing with the AIDS epidemic (Brandt, 1988).

The third reason for the failure of leadership and the absence of national policy is a lack of resources, both financial and human (Kirp & Bayer, 1992; Shilts, 1987). The epidemic hit when Reagan was initiating a wholesale assault on the American welfare state. As Kirp and Bayer argue, the Reagan administration:

> . . . was encouraging political and social forces committed to a traditional and restrictive vision of moral norms in public life. Consequently, at a time when vigorous federal action was demanded to deal effectively with the new epidemic— when a massive infusion of resources for research and prevention efforts would be called for, when great sums for social and medical services would be needed,

and when a capacity to break with the anti-gay trends in American culture would be required—the administration consistently minimized the issue and denigrated those who urged a more activist national role. (Kirp & Bayer, p. 9, 1992)

The American right pushed for a national political agenda that punished those who deservingly were dying from a disease they had brought upon themselves.

The failure of leadership is significant both at the domestic level and also globally. The United States was the nation where the disease was first publicized and where two thirds of the world's caseload outside of Africa can be found (Mann et. al., 1992). Policymakers in other nations have looked to America for examples of how to handle this epidemic; for the most part what they have been shown is how not to handle this epidemic. The failure to act responsibly in the face of the epidemic has had a resounding impact on the political and medical courses that the epidemic has taken. The response has been inadequate and uncoordinated. What success there has been has mostly been at the local level in cities such as San Francisco, Los Angeles, and New York. The ineffectiveness of the national government is symbolized by the failure of any administration to implement any significant number of the Presidential Commission's recommendations.

Policy leadership is as important as financial support; in spite of the late influx of funds, the appointment of the AIDS coordinator (commonly referred to as the AIDS Czar) Kristine Gebbie in August 1993, there is still inadequate government mobilization, complacency, and lack of coordinated and strategic planning in the fight against AIDS. In spite of President Clinton's rhetoric of supportive leadership on AIDS, his administration is no different from its predecessors. Perhaps Gebbie's appointment in August 1993 and resignation in July 1994 is the best reflection of how the Clinton administration is carrying out its AIDS policies. Gebbie's appointment was lost amid Clinton's first controversy: gays in the military. To compound this Gebbie was a candidate that was chosen not for what she could accomplish on AIDS, but for what she would do for Clinton. It was argued she would not hurt him. The role of the AIDS Czar was to be one of image, that the administration was doing something to stop AIDS. Thus, the job of the Czar was not to be a policymaker, but rather a facilitator; someone to act as a liaison between agencies. It was a pure exercise in public relations on the part of the Clinton administration.

THE DELIVERY OF PUBLIC HEALTH IN A CAPITALIST ECONOMY

There are inborn incongruities in the delivery of public health services in an economy such as America's. The ruling class has conflicting interests. On the one hand healthy workers are needed to maintain production, and the working class wants public health care. Everyone is susceptible to the same diseases. On the other hand, there are costs in providing public health. On one level these are financial, so often the ruling class does too little too late. On another level, the costs are political. This is the biggest problem that AIDS poses for capitalism.

A proper campaign against AIDS would require an open discussion of sexual practices of every variety with free condoms being openly available. However, all of this goes against the ruling class's political need to reinforce the control and distortion of sexuality within the lives of the working class (Foucault, 1979; German, 1989). There are several reasons for this. The first is the family. Capitalism needs the family economically. The primary costs of taking care of the young, the old, and the disabled all fall upon the families of wage earners, not upon the state or capital. If capitalism is to defend the family in its present form, that means attacking all forms of sexual activity that take place outside the family (German, 1989).

But the ruling class also needs, at some level, the compliant acquiescence of the working class to the system. If the simple economic interests of workers push them into struggle with capital, all the more important for the ruling class to reinforce prejudices and bigotry within the minds of the working class. It is in the interests of the ruling class to prevent individuals from taking conscious control of their own sex. A woman who is ashamed of an abortion is scared and lessened. A homosexual who dares not come out of the "closet" is frightened and diminished. A woman who insists upon condoms is taking control of one part of her life. Sexual lives are not hermetically sealed from political and working lives. Individuals are simultaneously lovers, workers, and political beings. Any increase in confidence and control in an individual's private life will have repercussions upon their public life. Sex and work are basic human needs, but under capitalism both are controlled, mystified, alienated, and drained of pleasure, satisfaction, and love. For there is a constant struggle over work and sex for a sense of liberation.

Ronald Reagan was part of a larger, political agenda of the American Right that had several stages. First, organized labor was assailed. This was achieved by breaking the air traffic controller's strike and inducing union leaders into "give back" wage cut contracts. Second, social services of all kinds were attacked. Thus, the massive cuts on health programs, education, and welfare. Third, the politics of the 1960s were reversed. This meant an attack on the "Vietnam Syndrome," both internationally and domestically. Within America it also meant a concerted attack on all movements and ideology from those years. Thus, the African American image was changed from civil rights protester to urban criminal, drug addict, and pusher. And it also meant denigrating gay liberation. Gays were perceived to be part of a "leftist" conspiracy aimed at undermining the American way of life; a misperception that is based upon a failure to see that homosexuality spans every socioeconomic and ideological cleavage of American society.

AIDS was an opportunity for the New Right; it was a vehicle for the reassertion of family values, of chastity, and fidelity, and for the denunciation and segregation of sexual deviance (Watney, 1988). As Weeks (1988, pp. 12–13) argues, AIDS provided the opportunity to undermine the changes of the sixties and seventies. It was a yardstick by which to measure the "supposed" decline of moral standards. So for its first five years Reagan's administration did nothing about AIDS. Any money for AIDS would mean less money for already existing programs facing already existing cuts (Shilts, 1987). In 1987, with the spread of the disease at crisis level, money appropriated by Congress was not spent (Kramer, 1990).

This was not serious only for Americans; the United States is the center of basic scientific information in almost every area of knowledge. If the resources were to be mobilized to understand and cure the disease, they were going to be mobilized in American labs and universities. In Great Britain, under Reagan's greatest ally, Margaret Thatcher, there was similar government indifference and even more cuts in scientific spending. The result in Britain has been almost no scientific AIDS research (Street & Weale, 1992).

At the core of capitalist society is industrial production and a relationship of power between men and women. This relationship of power permeates through and conditions the whole of society. It shapes every institution. The spread of HIV and AIDS and the failure to find a cure is the direct cause of capitalism's inability to produce for human need. The disease also spreads because sexual repression is basic to the perpetuation of capitalist society. History has shown that pestilence, war, and famine are inherent in a system governed by profit and not by human need.

CONCLUSION

This study has attempted to evaluate the American political system's response to AIDS since 1981 at the federal level. Within such an analysis, the focus has been on HIV/AIDS as a pandemic that is out of control, on the demographics of the disease, and on the problems of public health provision in a capitalist economy. The AIDS epidemic calls for not only an ardent reaction, but also a highly political one. The epidemic is a human catastrophe that demands outrage and remorse. It is also a political tragedy because successive presidential administrations since 1981 have dealt with AIDS with neglect despite well-meaning rhetoric. There has been legislation passed to combat discrimination against those individuals who are HIV positive or who have AIDS. However, this is insufficient to battle the political and social ravages of the epidemic.

The argument that capitalism has exacerbated the rampage of the epidemic, may seem harsh and somewhat suspect to many. Indeed, some would argue that this conclusion enables individuals to deny sorrow, to direct individual anguish into abstract wrath, to blame the system rather then their own behavior. It does not make sense to blame capitalism if one thinks of it as simply an economic system. The argument is that capitalism is not solely an economic system, it is also a social system with heavy social costs and burdens for those classes who do not control the means of production and the resources of society.

There has been no attempt to look at particular policies that government has enacted at the federal, state and local levels, but rather the focus has been on the failure of leadership at the national level to formulate and implement a national policy for meeting the demands of the epidemic. The appropriation of funds for AIDS in the federal budget is not a policy, although it could be argued to be a strategy.

The significance of AIDS is not who is affected, but that anyone should get it at all; it is not about someone being high risk, but that we place blame on the affected because they are already hated or feared; it is not about how it is transmitted, but that it should be prevented; it is not on the numbers who are infected or who have died, but how close it is to everyone. The further an individual thinks the disease is from them, the longer the question of the epidemic's actual significance for society will be put off.

The ultimate importance of AIDS is that it should make us question a health care system where thirty seven million Americans are without coverage and where another thirty five million have insufficient coverage (Davis & Rowland, 1991; Fain, 1993; Smith, 1993; Strauss, 1991). The United States has a three-tiered medical system that is reflective of the class structure perpetuated by capitalism. Indeed AIDS has increased the existing contradictions of the American health care system, and these same contradictions will make the system's response to the disease less and less effective. As Hunt (1988, p. 23) argues the AIDS epidemic is a crisis grafted upon a crisis that has sharply brought out all of the incongruities within the medical system.

Finally, for those individuals who feel that this virus does not discriminate against economic systems and thus, cite the presence of the virus in the Eastern bloc during communist rule, it is the contention of this author that such states were in fact state capitalist nations (Cliff, 1988; Harman, 1988; Hore, 1991). Under state capitalism the conditions and dynamics of the epidemic were similar to those that occurred in the United States under capitalism.

REFERENCES

Altman, D. (1986). *AIDS in the Mind of America.* Garden City, NY: Anchor Books.

Arno, P.S. (Nov 1986). The non-profit sectors response to the AIDS epidemic. *American Journal of Public Health,* pp. 42–47.

Arno, P.S., & K.L. Feiden. (1993). *Against the Odds.* New York: Harper Perennial.

Aukerman, G.F. (1991). Access to health care for the uninsured. *Journal of the American Medical Association,* pp. 2856–58.

Brandt, A.M. (1988). AIDS in historical perspective: four cases from the history of sexually transmitted diseases. *American Journal of Public Health,* 78: pp. 367–71.

Buehler, J.W. (Oct 1990). Impact of the human immunodeficiency virus epidemic on mortality trends in young men. *American Journal of Public Health,* pp. 1080–85.

Centers for Disease Control and Prevention. (1994). *HIV/AIDS Surveillance Report,* 6: p. 1.

Cliff, T. (1988). *State Capitalism in Russia.* London: Verso.

Cockerell, C.J., & G. Nary. (1991). AIDS discrimination and access to health care. *AIDS Patient Care,* 2: pp. 2–8.

Crimp, D., & A. Rolston. (1990). *AIDS Demographics.* Seattle: Vantage Press.

Cropley, N. E. (1994). The American "right" to health care—an idea whose time has come. *Golden State University Law Review,* 2: pp. 681–694.

Davis, K., & D. Rowland. (Spring 1991). The rights and duties of health care providers. *AIDS & Public Policy Journal,* pp. 31–39.

Desvarieux, M., & J.W. Pape. (1991). HIV and AIDS in Haiti. *AIDS Care,* 3: pp. 271–80.

Duesberg, P. (Feb 1989). Human immunodeficiency virus and acquired immunodeficiency syndrome: correlation but not causation. Memo Paper, *National Academy of Sciences.*

Ehrhardt, A.A. (Nov 1992.) Trends in sexual behavior and the HIV pandemic. *American Journal of Public Health,* pp. 1459–61.

Epstein, S. (April/June 1991). Democratic science? AIDS activism and the contested construction of knowledge. *Socialist Review,* pp. 35-61.

Fain, R. (Spring 1993). What we need is health care. *Foundation for the Study of Independent Social Ideas,* pp. 146–48.

Fauci, A. (1988). The human immunodeficiency virus. *Science,* 239: pp. 617–22.

Foucault, M. (1979). *History of Sexuality, Vol. 1.* London: Allen Lane.

Freudenberg, N. (Summer 1990). AIDS prevention in the U.S.: lessons from the first decade. *International Journal of Health Services,* pp. 589–99.

German, L. (1989). *Sex, Class and Socialism.* London: Verso.

Gladwell, M. (June 1993). Only Select. *The New Republic,* pp. 21–27.

Gostin, L. (1989). The politics of AIDS. *Ohio State Law Journal,* pp. 1039–49.

Grutsch, J.F., & A.D.J. Robertson. (March 1986). The coming of AIDS: it didn't start with homosexuals and it won't end with them. *American Spectator,* pp. 33–42.

Harman, C. (1988). *Class Struggle in Eastern Europe, 1945–1983,* 3rd ed. London: Verso.

Herek, G.M., & J.P. Capitanio. (April 1993). Public relations to AIDS in the U.S. *American Journal of Public Health,* pp. 574–77.

Hore, C. (1991). *The Road to Tiananman Square.* London: Verso.

Huber, G., & B. Schnerder. (May 1992). The Social Context of AIDS. *AIDS,* pp. 145–61.

Hunt, C.W. (Jan 1988). AIDS and capitalist medicine. *Monthly Review,* pp. 11–25.

Hurowitz, J.C. (1993). Sounding board toward a social policy for health. *New England Journal of Medicine,* 32: pp. 130–33.

Kalichman, S.C. (Oct 1992). The disclosure of celebrity HIV infection: its effects on public attitudes. *American Journal of Public Health,* pp. 1374–76.

Kirp, D., & R. Bayer. (1992). *AIDS in the Industrialized Democracies.* New Brunswick, N.J.: Rutgers University Press.

Kramer, L. (1990). *Reports from the Holocaust: The Making of an AIDS Activist.* London: Penguin.

Mann, J.M., D.J.M. Tarantola, & T.W. Netler, eds. (1992). *AIDS in the World.* Cambridge, Mass.: Harvard University Press.

Manuel, C. (Spring 1991). AIDS: The rights and duties of health care providers. *AIDS & Public Policy Journal,* pp. 31–39.

Maticka-Tyndale, E. (Aug 1992). Social construction of HIV transmission and prevention among heterosexual young adults. *Social Problems,* pp. 238–52.

Mcguire, J.F. (1989). AIDS: the community based response. *AIDS*, 5: pp. 279–82.

Novello, A.C. (1991). Women and HIV infection. *Journal of the American Medical Association*, 265: pp. 1805–20.

Palca, J. (1991). The sobering geography of AIDS. *Science*, 252: pp. 372–76.

Patton, C. (1990). *Inventing AIDS*. New York: Basic Books.

Payne, F.J. (June 1992). Community based case management of HIV disease. *American Journal of Public Health*, pp. 893–901.

Safyer, A.W., & G. Spies-Karotkin (1988). The biology of AIDS. *Health & Social Work*, 5: pp. 251–56.

Shayne, V.T. (Mar 1991). Double victims: poor women and AIDS. *Women & Health*, pp. 21–57.

Shilts, R. (1987). *And the Band Played On*. New York: St. Martins Press.

Smith, R.B. (Mar/Apr 1993). Health care reform now! *Social Science & Modern Society*, pp. 56–65.

Somerville, M.A., & A.J. Orkin. (1989). Human rights, discrimination, and AIDS concepts and issues. *AIDS*, 3 (suppl. 1): pp. S283–87.

Strauss, A. (July/Aug 1991). AIDS and health care deficiency. *Society*, pp. 63–73.

Street, J., & A. Weale. (1992). British policy making in a hermetically sealed system, in Kirp & Bayer, eds., *AIDS in the Industrialized Democracies*, pp. 185–225. New Brunswick, N.J.: Rutgers University Press.

Stuntzner-Gibson, D. (1991). Women and HIV disease: an emerging social crisis. *Social Work*, 36: pp. 22–27.

Wachter, R.M. (Jan 1992). AIDS, activism and the politics of health. *The New England Journal of Medicine*, pp. 128–132.

Watney, S. (1988). AIDS, moral panic theory and homophobia in Aggleton, P., and Homans, H., (eds.). *Social Aspects of AIDS*. Lewes, Sussex: Falmer Press.

Weeks, J. (1988). Love in a cold climate, in Aggleton P., and Homans, H., eds. *Social Aspects of AIDS*.

2

The Politics of Prevention and Neglect

Ronald Bayer

. . . . The remarkable advances in the biomedical realm and the formulation of public policies designed to limit the spread of human immunodeficiency virus (HIV) infection and protect the rights of those who are infected or at risk of infection stand as singular accomplishments. Their success is all the more striking because it has come as a consequence of intense political conflict, spurred by the demands of those who have borne the burden of disease and their allies. But these achievements also set the stage for new controversies in public health. The central political and ethical question of privacy that provided the core theme of political debate in the epidemic's first phase has now been joined, although not displaced, by that of equity.

Recent clinical developments are critical to an understanding of the evolving political debates about AIDS and public health. While it is still too soon to speak of AIDS itself as a chronic disease, HIV infection will increasingly require the long-term clinical management associated with such conditions. As a consequence, identifying those who are infected has become even more crucial. No longer is the question before public health officials solely a matter of preventing infection. Increasingly, providing the million or more infected Americans with appropriate clinical supervision has become a higher priority. Within this changed context, screening, reporting, and partner noti-

Bayer, Ronald. "The Politics of Prevention and Neglect," from "AIDS: The Politics of Prevention," as appeared in *Health Affairs* (Spring 1991), pp. 87–97. Reprinted by permission of Project HOPE, The People-to-People Health Foundation, Health Affairs, 7500 Old Georgetown Road, Suite 600, Bethesda, MD 20814, 301–656–7401.

fication—issues that figured so prominently in the early controversies over AIDS prevention—have provoked fresh debates about the appropriate role of the state. The traditional approaches of public health officials to epidemic disease, so vigorously challenged in the early and mid–1980s, have found new support from those who had recently considered these approaches inadequate or ethically unacceptable.

HIV ANTIBODY TESTING AND EARLY INTERVENTION

No issue has consumed more attention in the disputes over public policy and AIDS than the use of the antibody test to identify those infected with HIV. Out of these debates emerged a broad consensus, often codified in state statutes, that testing should be conducted only with the informed voluntary and specific consent of individuals. Despite that standard and the carefully defined, though always contested, exceptions to its scope, many clinicians and hospitals undertook surreptitious testing of patients, justifying their practices by the belief that the protection of health care workers and sound diagnostic work required such screening.[1]

In mid–1989, clinical trials revealed the efficacy of early therapeutic intervention in slowing the course of illness in asymptomatic but infected persons and in preventing the occurrence of *Pneumocystis carinii* pneumonia. At this point, the political debate about testing underwent a fundamental change. Groups such as Project Inform in San Francisco and the Gay Men's Health Crisis in New York City began to encourage those they had formerly warned against testing to determine whether or not they were infected.[2] Physicians pressed more vigorously for the "return of AIDS to the medical mainstream" so that testing might be routinely done under conditions of presumed consent.[3] Public health officials (most notably in New York and New Jersey, which had borne so much of the burden of AIDS) launched aggressive testing campaigns.

Although physicians and public health officials have typically avoided the language of compulsion, stressing instead routine testing, the threat of coercion continues to loom before gay activists, their liberal political allies, and proponents of civil liberties. So too has the risk of increased stigma and discrimination within the context of medical institutions.

As early therapeutic intervention continues to show promise, the alliances forged in the first phase of the epidemic have begun to unravel. Nowhere is this clearer than in the emergence of a powerful movement, supported by obstetricians and pediatricians, for the routine screening of pregnant women who could transmit HIV to their offspring and the mandatory screening of infants at high risk for infection. In the case of the former, the public health practice of testing for syphilis and hepatitis B serves as a model. In the latter instance, the wide-scale and broadly accepted tradition of screening for congenital conditions such as phenylketonuria (PKU) provides the standard. The promise—with little evidentiary base—that early intervention might protect the fetus or at least enhance the life prospects of babies at risk for HIV infection has begun to override ethical concerns about the coercive identification of infected women, most of whom are black or Hispanic, as well as about the potential burdens of exclusion from housing, social services, and health care itself that might be imposed on those so identified.

REPORTING, CONTACT TRACING, AND CONFIDENTIALITY

The erosion of the alliance that had resisted the application of traditional public health practices to AIDS can be seen also in the shifting trends on the issue of reporting the names of those infected with HIV to confidential public health department registries. Gay groups and their allies had fiercely resisted such reporting requirements because of concerns about privacy and confidentiality. Public health officials in areas with large numbers of AIDS cases also opposed reporting because it might leave people less willing to seek voluntary HIV testing and counseling. As a consequence, reporting requirements had become policy in only a few states. By the late 1980s, fissures had begun to appear in the alliance opposing named reporting in those states where the prevalence of HIV infection was high and where gay communities were well organized.

In June 1989, Stephen Joseph, then commissioner of health in New York City, told the Fifth International Conference on AIDS in Montreal that the prospect of early clinical intervention necessitated "a shift toward a disease control approach to HIV infection along the lines of classic tuberculosis practices."[4] Central to such an approach would be the "reporting of seropositives" to assure effective clinical follow-up and "more aggressive contact tracing." Joseph's proposals opened a debate that was only temporarily settled by the defeat of New York's Mayor Edward Koch in his 1989 bid for reelection. When newly elected Mayor David Dinkins selected Woodrow Myers, formerly commissioner of health in Indiana, to replace Joseph, his appointment was almost aborted, in part because he had supported named reporting.[5] The festering debate was ended only by a political decision on the part of the mayor, who had drawn heavily on support within the gay community, to stand by his appointment while promising that there would be no named reporting.

In New Jersey, which shares with New York City a relatively high level of HIV infection, the commissioner of health also supported named reporting, but the politics surrounding the issue were very different. There, both houses of the state legislature endorsed without dissent a confidentiality statute that included named reporting of cases of HIV infection.[6] New Jersey simply exemplified a national trend. For, although at the end of 1989 only nine states required named reporting without any provision for anonymity, states increasingly were adopting policies that required reporting in at least some circumstances.[7] And always the arguments were the same. New therapeutic possibilities provided the warrant for reestablishing a standard of traditional public health practice.

Ironically, pressure to extend the provision of Medicaid coverage for early treatment and to expand government-funded clinics to treat those with HIV infection will inevitably result in the creation of records on growing numbers of infected individuals, regardless of whether states adopt mandatory reporting requirements. The move toward early clinical intervention then is incompatible with the preservation of anonymity. As a result, creating and enforcing regimes to protect the rights of infected persons from acts of discrimination will become even more important than in the epidemic's first years. In this context, not only state-level protections for individuals with HIV infection will be crucial. More important will be the implementation and enforcement of the Americans with Disabilities Act, legislation that explicitly includes those with HIV infection among the protected class covered by the enactment.

The move toward named reporting was linked only in part to the argument that state health departments needed the names of individuals to assure adequate clinical follow-up. Public health officials also asserted that effective contact tracing, now more critical than ever because of the need for early clinical intervention, could be undertaken only if those with HIV infection, but who were not yet diagnosed as having AIDS, could be interviewed. Despite its central and well-established role in venereal disease control, the notification of sexual and needle-sharing partners in the context of AIDS had been a source of ongoing conflict between gay groups and civil liberties organizations on the one hand, and public health officials who had proposed such a strategy in the early years of the epidemic on the other. This notification was always predicated on the willingness of those with sexually transmitted diseases to provide public health workers with the names of their partners in exchange for a promise of anonymity. A standard disease control measure, it had been viewed by AIDS activists as a threat to confidentiality and as a potentially coercive intervention. Indeed, opponents of contact tracing typically denounced it as "mandatory."

With time and a better understanding of how contact tracing functioned in the context of sexually transmitted diseases (STDs), some of the most vocal opponents of tracing yielded their principled opposition at least in private meetings and discussions and instead centered their concerns on the cost of so labor-intensive an intervention. Nevertheless, support for voluntary contact tracing was ultimately to come from the Institute of Medicine and the National Academy of Sciences, the Presidential Commission on the HIV Epidemic, the American Bar Association, and the American Medical Association (AMA).[8] Indeed, it was the AMA's support for tracing, justified by then executive vice-president James Sammons as having "the potential in the heterosexual society to substantially reduce the proliferation and spread of AIDS," that provided the grounds for the group's support for mandatory HIV reporting.[9]

The U.S. Centers for Disease Control (CDC) has been most active in pressing for the adoption of contact tracing programs at the state level, where all such programs are organized and funded.[10] Critically involved in the training of STD workers and in the funding of local venereal disease programs, CDC had from the outset urged the adoption of this standard public health approach to AIDS and HIV infection. In February 1988, the federal agency took on a more aggressive posture, making the adoption of partner notification by the states a condition for the receipt of funds from its HIV Prevention Program.[11] Despite such pressure, the response on the part of the states has been variable. States most heavily burdened by AIDS have continued to favor programs that encourage infected individuals to notify their own partners. Of the states that stressed the role of professional public health workers—the "provider referral" model—most have tended to have relatively modest AIDS case counts.[12] Thus, local epidemiological factors as well as political forces have continued to influence the course of public health policy.

In part, both the early and the lingering resistance to partner notification can be explained by the confusion of the standard public health approach to STD control with policies and practices that are rooted in a very different tradition, entailing a "duty to warn" or protect those who might be threatened by individuals with communicable conditions. When such warnings have been deemed appropriate and legal, they have occurred without the consent of the index case and typically have involved the revelation of the identity of the threatening party.

The early and strict confidentiality rules surrounding HIV screening and medical records in many states all but precluded physicians from warning individuals placed at risk by their sexual and needle-sharing partners. In recent years, the recognition that such limitations placed physicians in a position that sometimes violated professional ethical norms, the realization that some patients could pose a grave threat to unsuspecting partners, and the increasing importance of early therapeutic intervention have led to modifications of early confidentiality restrictions. Such modifications were often opposed on principled grounds by those who believed that physician/patient communications should never be violated and by those who argued that such breaches of confidentiality would have the counterproductive consequence of reducing patient candor, thus limiting the capacity of clinicians to effectively counsel and persuade individuals who might harm their partners. Yet they have been given strong support in a number of state legislatures and by the AMA and the Association of State and Territorial Health Officials.[13] As of 1990, no state had imposed upon physicians a duty to warn unsuspecting partners. But about a dozen had adopted legislation granting physicians a "privilege to warn or inform," thus freeing physicians from liability for either warning or not warning those at risk.[14]

The question of how to respond to individuals whose behavior represented a threat to unknowing partners inevitably provoked continued discussion of the public health tradition of imposing restrictions on liberty in the name of communal welfare. Although all efforts to bring AIDS within the scope of state quarantine statutes have been fiercely opposed, more than twenty states did so between 1987 and 1990.[15] States typically used the occasion to modernize their disease control laws to reflect contemporary constitutional standards that detail procedural guarantees, and to require that restrictions on freedom represent the "least restrictive alternative" available to achieve a "compelling state interest."

With the exception of the few notable cases that have received press attention, there is no well-documented review of the extent to which newly revised quarantine statutes have been applied to the AIDS epidemic. There are, however, data to suggest that the power vested in public health officials by such laws has been used more often to warn than to incarcerate those whose behavior has posed a risk of HIV transmission. But, in any case, the numbers have been small. It is clear, therefore, that the enactment of revised quarantine laws has been responsive to political pressures and the belief in the efficacy of symbolic bulwarks.

The enactment of statutes criminalizing behavior linked to the spread of AIDS has paralleled political receptivity to laws extending the authority of public health officials to control individuals whose behavior posed a risk of HIV transmission. Such use of the criminal law, broadly endorsed by the Presidential Commission on the HIV Epidemic in 1988, called upon a tradition of state enactments that made the knowing transmission of venereal disease a crime.[16] Though they almost never were enforced, these older laws served as a rationale for new legislative initiatives. Between 1987 and 1989, twenty states enacted such statutes, most of which defined the proscribed acts as felonies, despite the fact that older statutes typically treated knowing transmission as a misdemeanor.[17] Recent congressional action to increase federal support for local AIDS initiatives has conditioned the receipt of funds on the existence of state authority to prosecute individuals who knowingly expose unsuspecting persons to HIV.[18] As important, aggressive prosecutors have relied on laws defining assaultive behavior and attempted murder to bring indictments, even in the absence of AIDS–specific legislation.

Any effort to determine to what extent prosecutions of HIV–related acts have occurred must confront the difficulty of monitoring the activity of local courts when there is neither a guilty verdict nor an appeal to a higher state tribunal. One survey, relying on newspaper accounts as well as official court reports, estimated that 50–100 prosecutions had been initiated involving acts as diverse as spitting, biting, blood splattering, blood donation, and sexual intercourse with an unsuspecting partner.[19] Though small in number, these cases have drawn great attention. In many cases, prosecution has been unsuccessful. Nevertheless, punishment for some of those found guilty has been unusually harsh.

PREVENTION AND BEHAVIOR CHANGE

Whatever the allure of such measures and of the rediscovery of traditional public health approaches in the effort to combat the spread of HIV infection, it has remained clear that the future course of the AIDS epidemic will be determined by the creation of a social and institutional milieu within which radical voluntary changes in behavior can occur and be sustained. Educational campaigns and counseling programs, most effectively undertaken by groups linked to the populations at risk, have remained the centerpiece of that preventive effort. Such efforts are, however, still limited by moralistic trends in American society, especially by those reflecting abhorrence of homosexuality.

The most striking failure in the preventive realm, however, is rooted in the unwillingness to commit the resources necessary to treat drug abuse. The dimensions of that failure were underscored in the 1988 preliminary report of the Presidential Commission on the HIV Epidemic.[20] In its first report to President George Bush issued in December 1989, the National Commission on Acquired Immune Deficiency Syndrome underscored the continuing failure. As did its predecessor, the National Commission on AIDS—chaired by June Osborn, a well-known critic of federal AIDS policy, and vice-chaired by David Rogers, a persistent voice for increased federal support to the cities most severely affected by the epidemic—called for the availability of treatment "on request" for all drug users.[21]

Concern about budgetary deficits, ten years of ideological opposition to welfare state–like programs by conservative national administrations, and the absence of a strong political constituency capable of effectively clamoring for the needs of the underclass have resulted in a politics of neglect. It is in this context that opposition or suspicion on the part of black and Hispanic community leaders to the halfway measures of needle exchange and education about the use of bleach to cleanse drug injection equipment must be understood.[22] In the absence of a strong commitment to treatment, such measures appear to write off the needs of the poor. Thus, there has emerged an alliance of the moralistic right and those who speak in the name of the dispossessed. The first black commissioner of health in New York City, acting at the behest of the city's first black mayor, terminated a small and politically hobbled needle exchange program soon after assuming office.[23] More stunning, he sought to cancel a small municipal contract that funded a community-based group to provide drug users with bleach and education about how to sterilize injection equipment.[24]

The failure to fund drug abuse services was but a portion of a much deeper problem: the failure of the federal government to plan for and assist those localities that were compelled to bear the burden of providing care for large numbers of patients with AIDS. The dimensions of that failure would become even starker with the 1989 announcements on the potential benefits of early therapeutic intervention for people infected with HIV.

THE CHALLENGE OF AN EQUITABLE RESPONSE TO AIDS

Here then was a paradox not new to the American health care system. Extraordinary advances in medicine must inevitably confront the social reality of the most inequitable system of medical care among advanced democratic societies. Could such a health care system meet the challenge of providing between 500,000 and 1,000,000 persons, many of whom are impoverished, with the outpatient clinical services and the expensive drugs they would require? Would it be possible for an unjust health care system to fashion a just response to those infected with HIV? Before these questions, the earlier important debates about discrimination by private medical insurers paled.

Emergency federal programs to assist the states in paying the cost of zidovudine, or AZT, for those without insurance, Medicaid reimbursement policies, and a host of patchwork programs in the states provided some relief but were clearly inadequate.[25] In its December 1989 report to the president, the National Commission on AIDS warned that medical breakthroughs would "mean little unless the health care system can incorporate them and make then accessible to people in need."[26] The existence of a medically disenfranchised class meant that, for many, access to care was almost solely through the 'emergency room door of one of the few hospitals in the community that treats people with HIV infection and AIDS." This is hardly the foundation for the kind of care HIV infection will require in the 1990s.

The situation that prevailed in New York City, the epicenter of the American AIDS epidemic, was extreme because of the existence of a number of concurrent sociomedical and economic crises, including drug abuse, homelessness, and dire fiscal conditions. Nevertheless, it revealed how a failure to plan effectively and commit sufficient resources, itself a consequence of federal default, could have catastrophic results, not only for those with HIV–related disorders and the poor—so dependent on publicly provided medical services—but for the system of health care more generally.

It was not too soon to start thinking of worst-case scenarios.[27] Shortages would impose the need for rationing, and in the political economy of a city such as New York, competition among the desperate would ensue. In what Bruce Vladek has termed the "calculus of misery," it would become increasingly necessary to choose between AIDS cases and the frail elderly for admission to nursing homes; between single adults with AIDS and homeless families with young children for access to newly renovated apartments; between homeless persons dying of AIDS and children for access to transitional shelter; and between HIV–infected pregnant women and women not yet infected for admission to drug abuse treatment programs.

The looming crisis in health care for those with HIV disease set the stage for congressional action in 1990 that could scarcely have been imagined a short time earlier. This action was the fruit of dogged efforts by AIDS activists, their allies, and some political leaders from the cities and states that had borne the disproportionate share of AIDS cases. Early in 1990, Sen. Edward Kennedy (D-MA), the exemplar of Democratic party liberalism, and Sen. Orrin Hatch (R-UT), a Republican whose stance on abortion and other social issues casts him in the role of a conservative, jointly sponsored legislation— the Ryan White Comprehensive AIDS Resources Emergency Act of 1990— that would provide a major infusion of federal assistance to those localities most severely burdened by AIDS. As the government had responded to natural disasters, the Ryan White bill asked it to respond to the medical disaster of AIDS: "The Human Immunodeficiency Virus constitutes a crisis as devastating as an earthquake, flood or drought. Indeed, the death toll of the unfolding AIDS tragedy is already a hundredfold greater than any natural disaster to strike our nation in this century."[28]

As remarkable as was the joint sponsorship of this legislation, which promised to provide $2.9 billion over five years in a complex political formula to the cities and states most severely struck by AIDS, was the overwhelming support the legislation received in the Senate, where the vote was 95 to 4.[29] When similar legislation with even greater resource commitments was voted on by the House of Representatives, the vote was 408 to 14.[30]

However late in coming, this legislation represented on both symbolic and practical levels an important act of national solidarity. But the hopes of early summer were dashed by fall as Congress, confronted with a severe budgetary crisis, slashed funds for the Ryan White Act. What allocations will be made in successive years cannot be foretold. It is certain, however, that such an emergency act cannot be a substitute for the fundamental change in the organization and financing of health care in the United States that will be required for the chronic management of the medical and social needs of all HIV–infected persons at a moment when so many other medical needs of the nation's poor remain unmet.

Conventionally, the public health emphasis on prevention and the clinical commitment to caring for the sick have been viewed as conceptually distinct; they compete in the day-to-day struggle over limited resources. With the rapid development of therapies for HIV disease, it has become clear that prevention and care are joined in a critical way. Public health officials have used the occasion of new therapeutic prospects as a justification for rethinking preventive policies adopted in the epidemic's first years. But the prospect of new therapies is not enough. They must be available to those who need them if lives are to be prolonged and if the public health goal of preventing the further spread of HIV infection is to be achieved. The possibility of engaging those with HIV infection in ongoing clinical care provides a crucial opportunity to sustain behavioral change where it has occurred and to encourage and support such change where it has not. A failure to provide care and counseling, especially to the poor among whom intravenous drug use plays so critical a role in HIV transmission, will entail both a sentence of needlessly shortened life and a lost opportunity to intervene in the epidemic's epidemiological course.

NOTES

1. Centers for Disease Control, "CDC Estimates of HIV Prevalence and Projected AIDS Cases: Summary of a Workshop, October 3–November 1989," *Morbidity and Mortality Weekly Report* (23 February 1990): 110–119.

2. *PI Perspective* (San Francisco: Project Inform, April 1988), 7; and *The New York Times*, 16 August 1989, 1.

3. F.S. Rhame and D.A. Maki, "The Case for Wide Use of Testing for HIV Infection," *The New England Journal of Medicine* 320, no. 19 (1989): 1248–1254.

4. S.C. Joseph, "Remarks at the V International Conference on AIDS," Montreal, Quebec, 5 June 1989 (mimeo).

5. *The New York Times*, 19 January 1990, B-1.

6. *Newark Star Ledger*, 5 January 1990.

7. Intergovernmental Health Policy Project, "HIV Reporting in the States," *Intergovernmental AIDS Reports* (November–December 1989).

8. National Academy of Sciences, Institute of Medicine, *Confronting AIDS: Update 1988* (Washington, D.C.: National Academy Press, 1988), 82; *Report of the Presidential Commission on the Human Immunodeficiency Virus Epidemic* (Washington, D.C.: U.S. Government Printing Office, June 1988), 76; American Bar Association, AIDS Coordinating Committee, *ABA Policy on AIDS* (August 1989); and *American Medical News* (8–15 July 1988), 4.

9. *American Medical News* (8–15 July 1988), 4.

10. K. Toomey and W. Cates, "Partner Notification for the Prevention of HIV Infection," *AIDS* (Supplement 1, 1989): 557–562.

11. *Federal Register* 53, no. 24 (5 February 1988), 3554.

12. K. Toomey, "Partner Notification for HIV Prevention: Current State Programs and Policies in the United States" (paper presented at the V International Conference on AIDS, Montreal, Quebec, 7 June 1989).

13. Board of Trustees, American Medical Association, December 1989; and Association of State and Territorial Health Officials, National Association of County Health Officials, U.S. Conference of Local Health Officers, *Guide to Public Health Practice: HIV Partner Notification Strategies* (Washington, D.C.: Public Health Foundation, 1988).

14. Intergovernmental Health Policy Project, "1989 Legislative Overview," *Intergovernmental AIDS Reports* (January 1990): 3.

15. Based on a review of all AIDS–related legislation in the files of the Intergovernmental Health Policy Project, Washington, D.C.

16. *Report of the Presidential Commission on the HIV Epidemic,* 130–131.

17. Based on a review of all AIDS-related legislation in the files of the Intergovernmental Health Policy Project in Washington, D.C. See M.A. Field and K.M. Sullivan, "AIDS and the Criminal Law," *Law, Medicine and Health Care* (Summer 1987): 46–60.

18. Ryan White Comprehensive AIDS Resources Emergency Act, 1990, Section 2647.

19. L.O. Gostin, "The AIDS Litigation Project: A National Review of Court and Human Rights Commission Decisions, Part 1: The Social Impact of AIDS," *Journal of the American Medical Association* (11 April 1990): 1963.

20. *The New York Times* (25 February 1988), 1.

21. National Commission on Acquired Immune Deficiency Syndrome, "Report Number One" (Washington, D.C.: National Commission on AIDS, 5 December 1989).

22. H. Dalton, "AIDS in Black Face," *Daedalus* (Summer 1989): 205–227.

23. *The New York Times* (14 February 1990), B-1.

24. *American Medical News* (25 May 1990), 5.

25. Intergovernmental Health Policy Project, "AZT: Who Will Pay?" *Intergovernmental AIDS Reports* (May–June 1989): 4; and Intergovernmental Health Policy Project, "State Financing for AIDS: Options and Trends," *Intergovernmental AIDS Reports* (March–April 1990), 1–8, 12.

26. National Commission on AIDS, "Report Number One."

27. United Hospital Fund, "President's Letter" (New York: UHF, February 1990).

28. Sen. Edward M. Kennedy, letter, February 1990.

29. *The New York Times* (17 May 1990), B-10.

30. *The New York Times* (14 June 1990), B-9.

3

AIDS, Activism, and the Politics of Health

R. M. Wachter

The trends toward empowering patients and questioning scientific expertise antedated the epidemic of the acquired immunodeficiency syndrome (AIDS). As early as the late 1960s, observers noted an increase in the involvement of patients and their advocates in health care organization, provision, financing, and research.[1,2] Moreover, despite their traditional public emphasis on charitable activities, large health organizations like the American Cancer Society have long traditions of political advocacy.[3]

Nevertheless, the entry of AIDS activists into the health care scene has added a jarring new dimension to what was previously a genteel dialogue between patient advocates and clinicians, researchers, and policy makers. The activists' unprecedented modus operandi is a study in contrasts: street theater and intimidation on the one hand, detailed position papers and painstaking negotiation on the other. The effect has been to energize the fight against AIDS with an urgency that has translated into expedited drug approvals, lower prices for medications, and increased funding for AIDS research and care.[4]

The increasing influence of AIDS activists on health care decision making has not been universally praised, however. The movement is under attack for using militant tactics,[5,6] alienating natural allies such as physicians and scientists, and inadequately embracing the viewpoints of the diverse groups at risk for human immunodeficiency virus (HIV) infection and AIDS. Recent

From Wachter, R. M. "AIDS, Activism, and the Politics of Health," *The New England Journal of Medicine* (January 1992), pp. 128–133. Copyright © 1992, Massachusetts Medical Society. Reprinted by permission of The New England Journal of Medicine.

articles in the *Journal*[7,8] have argued that partly because of the activists' clout, the United States has adopted a policy of "HIV exceptionalism" that has compromised the public health response to the epidemic.

Now, a decade into the epidemic and five years after the founding of the AIDS Coalition to Unleash Power (ACT UP), the best-known activist group, it is appropriate to examine AIDS activism and its implications in the broad arena of health policy. In doing so, I will focus on four questions. First, what are the roots of AIDS activism, and why was the epidemic six years old before the movement crystallized? Second, why has AIDS activism been so successful in influencing policy? Third, what are the challenges faced by AIDS activists five years later? And finally, is this model of activism applicable to other diseases?

THE ROOTS OF AIDS ACTIVISM

To understand AIDS activism, one must examine the gay rights movement, because after a tragic period of hesitation, the one evolved directly from the other.

The modern gay-liberation movement began in 1969, when a police raid at the Stonewall Inn, a Greenwich Village bar, led to three days of rioting. During the 1970s the movement focused largely on sexual freedom, a focus that had two disastrous consequences when a new virus entered the gay community in the late 1970s. First, the promiscuity in the community facilitated the rapid spread of the new sexually transmitted pathogen. Second, when AIDS began to appear in the early 1980s, many members of the gay community resisted changes in sexual behavior and eschewed political militancy. Instead, groups such as the National Gay and Lesbian Task Force and the Gay Men's Health Crisis concentrated on caring for the ill and lobbying traditional targets (e.g., local officials) to oppose measures they saw as involving privacy issues, such as the closing of bathhouses and, later, the notification of partners.[9,10] The reasons for this early resistance to more aggressive forms of political activism included denial, a fear of losing the hard-won sexual freedom gained during the 1970s, and concern that a vigorous gay response to the epidemic would unleash a surge of homophobia.[4]

It was not until 1987, six years after the first AIDS cases were reported, that AIDS activism began in earnest, with a speech by author Larry Kramer to a gay group in Greenwich Village. Kramer warned his audience that most of those present would die unless they pressed the biomedical establishment to expedite the search for new AIDS treatments: "If what you're hearing doesn't rouse you to anger, fury, rage, and action, gay men will have no future here on earth."[11] Soon after the speech, ACT UP chapters began to form in cities around the country and, later, around the world.

Why did the AIDS activist movement finally coalesce in 1987? After all, some members of the gay community, including Kramer, had been arguing for increased militancy for years, arguments that had previously fallen on deaf ears.[9] What had changed? First, the gay community's fear that an active role in the epidemic would lead to an increase in homophobia had not materialized. In fact, polls showed an increase during the 1980s of nearly 50 percent in the percentage of adults who thought homosexual relations between consenting adults should be legal, a change that may have been fueled by sympathy for the gay community and respect born of its responsible handling of the epidemic.[12]

Second, the activist movement was stoked by the sheer dimensions of the epidemic. By 1987, more than 20,000 Americans, about three fourths of them gay, had died of the disease. It was now abundantly clear that the entire gay community was at risk; early hopes that the epidemic would be short-lived (like the outbreaks of legionnaires' disease and toxic shock syndrome a decade earlier) had long since been dismissed.

Third, the discovery of HIV in 1984 and the widespread availability of testing for the virus a year later provided tens of thousands of homosexual men with evidence of their impending mortality. Previously, the only people with such an intensely personal stake in finding a cure had been those with full-blown AIDS, who were often unable to engage in political warfare because of infirmity. People with newly diagnosed HIV seropositivity, who were usually asymptomatic, were imbued with a passion that comes only from seeing oneself at proximate risk.[13]

Finally, the discovery of HIV led to research on antiviral agents, some of which were only partway through the pipeline of federal research by 1987. If the government bureaucracy remained unchallenged, activists thought, the testing and approval of effective drugs would take years—years they simply did not have.

The confluence of these factors explains the origins of ACT UP and a new style of AIDS activism in 1987. In its first five years, the activist movement—sometimes praised, sometimes vilified, but always noticed—has permanently altered American health policy.

THE IMPACT OF AIDS ACTIVISM

The pressures brought to bear by AIDS activists on researchers, health officials, and the pharmaceutical industry have led to important changes in the course of the epidemic. Lobbying by HIV–infected people and their advocates led the Public Health Service to approve an expanded-access program, designed to make drugs available before the Food and Drug Administration had completed its approval process.[14] Similarly, pressure from activists led Burroughs Wellcome to lower the price of its antiretroviral drug zidovudine, or AZT.[15] Finally, activists are at least partly responsible for pressuring Congress into allocating a large sum of money, currently $1.7 billion a year, for AIDS research.

Why has the activist movement succeeded in promoting its agenda? The answer lies in the movement's organization and group consciousness, prefigured in the gay-rights movement. Gay people were deeply skeptical of the commitment by government (and society) to ensuring their well-being, a skepticism that translated into grass-roots mobilization and a unified focus. It is no coincidence that many members of ACT UP have embraced the theme of Malcolm X: "By any means necessary."[16]

The analogy to Malcolm X translates to strategy as well. Some civil-rights scholars attribute much of Dr. Martin Luther King, Jr.'s success to the radicalism of Malcolm X.[17,18] King, the argument goes, gained access to power brokers because they preferred to deal with him rather than with Malcolm X. The same argument explains some of the influence of radical AIDS groups, which has created room to operate not only for other, more temperate AIDS lobbying groups, but also for more moderate elements of the activist movement itself, such as ACT UP's Treatment and Data committees.

Access to policy makers would have been of only limited usefulness had the activists not included persons who were articulate, knowledgeable about the media, and able to use the levers of power. The largely middle-class gay communities of urban America contained sizable numbers of young, well-educated professionals able to seize an opportunity to make their points. In cities like New York and San Francisco, gays also represented large and powerful voting blocs with considerable political clout.

Finally, the targets of the activists—often scientists or medical policy makers within the bureaucracy of the Public Health Service—were relatively easy marks. Many came from liberal traditions and were sympathetic to the plight of people with AIDS. Unused to being at the center of a political maelstrom, some policy makers were easily intimidated by the activists. Moreover, health researchers and their patients are mutually interdependent. Researchers had to take seriously the threats of AIDS activists to sabotage drug trials, since the researchers required the participation of patients to complete their projects.

Because of all these factors, AIDS activism has enjoyed unprecedented success in shaping health policy. So much success, in fact, that in the past few years some have begun to ask whether AIDS is now getting more than its fair share of resources and whether it is being handled in a way contrary to the best interests of the public health.[19–21]

Beginning in 1989, some criticized the level of AIDS funding as being too generous as compared with funding for other serious illnesses.[22-23] For example, federal spending for AIDS was $1.6 billion in 1990, a year after 40,000 Americans died of the disease. During the same year, federal spending for cancer, a disease that killed 500,000 in 1989, was $1.5 billion, and spending for heart disease, which killed 750,000, was less than $1 billion.[30] Although spokespersons for the AIDS community often noted that AIDS resources did not come at the expense of other health care needs, in fact overall spending for health care research remained essentially fixed; it was self-evident that money spent on AIDS was money not spent on something else.[24] Similarly, the more hours that were used to expedite trials of antiviral agents and FDA evaluations, the fewer were available for other worthwhile pursuits.

In defending the recent priority given to AIDS, AIDS advocates say that AIDS is different from other diseases because it is epidemic and infectious— prompt action could contain the spread of the causative agent. It tends to strike the young, whereas cancer and heart disease tend to strike people in their 50s and 60s. AIDS has been centered in a dozen cities around the country and has ravaged their public health systems. Finally, progress on cancer and heart disease is seen as slow and incremental, whereas there is hope that AIDS—like polio before it—will one day be eradicated by a major scientific advance.[23] The point here is not that any particular allocation of resources is right or wrong, but rather that the success of AIDS activists demonstrated that decisions about the allocation of resources—even in health care—are inherently political and thus amenable to effective lobbying.

Before passing judgment on whether AIDS activists have indeed secured more than a fair share of resources for the HIV epidemic, we should ask whether activism would have been necessary had the initial response of government, the media, and the biomedical establishment been commensurate with the magnitude of the crisis.[9] Despite the activists' successes, the epidemic may still receive less money and attention than if it had struck mainstream American society with the same viciousness.

A second area cited by critics of AIDS advocacy involves the drug-approval process. AIDS activists, led by San Francisco's Project Inform, assert that they, not a federal agency, should be given the right to decide whether the benefits of an unproved but potentially effective new drug outweigh the risk for people suffering from fatal illnesses.[25] Activists challenged the FDA's regulatory authority directly by carrying out underground tests of new drugs, threatening to sabotage government-sponsored drug trials, and conducting massive demonstrations at FDA headquarters.[26] These tactics prompted the FDA to approve an expedited drug-approval process,[27] hailed as lifesaving by AIDS advocates but criticized as dangerous and costly by some in the scientific community. What, some researchers ask, will prevent the FDA from approving another Laetrile under its new policy, or even worse, another thalidomide?[28] Moreover, why should society subsidize the cost of medications prescribed simply because they might work?

Third, critics of the AIDS lobby point to its emphasis on developing new drugs to treat those already infected with HIV, as opposed to creating programs to prevent the spread of the virus. Politically, this bias can be explained by the lobby's origins in the gay activism of the 1970s. Homosexual men constituted the majority of people initially infected by HIV, and this relatively well-educated population quickly learned to practice prevention. Despite some recent reports of recidivism,[29] the low rate of new seroconversions among homosexual men has left that community concerned primarily with finding drugs to treat HIV infection and AIDS–related illnesses. Although AIDS activists have begun to pay more attention to prevention programs, such as needle exchange, their continued emphasis on cure over prevention has only limited relevance to other Americans, primarily heterosexual people of color in urban centers, who are still at high risk for HIV infection. This emphasis also troubles health care workers and policy makers in Africa and the rest of the developing world. In these countries, where the annual per capita health care budget is often less than $10, America's focus on determining the superiority of one antiviral agent over another seems cruelly wasteful and immaterial. Prevention is the only viable strategy.

Finally, critics of the activist movement, including many gay and HIV–infected people, condemn ACT UP's stridency and seeming willingness to deny free speech to such "enemies" as Dr. Louis Sullivan, secretary of the Department of Health and Human Services, who was shouted down at the Sixth International Conference on AIDS.[4] One gay editorialist expressed the community's misgivings as follows:

> There is a fine line between, on the one hand, street theater, civil disobedience, and the right to demonstrate, and on the other, mob behavior and brownshirting. . . . Many fear that the politics of anger is causing the community to abandon its commitment to the freedom of expression and the right to privacy, the two ideas used most often to support gay rights.[30,31]

AIDS activists defend their tactics, observing that their unprecedented access to medical decision makers—the opportunity to serve on advisory committees at the National Institutes of Health and the FDA and give major speeches at international AIDS conferences—was won largely because decision makers feared the disruption activists could create. Nevertheless, even supporters of the activist agenda are concerned that the tactics of harassment and intimidation may be generating an AIDS backlash, alienating members of mainstream society, and causing some researchers and pharmaceutical concerns to leave the choppy waters of AIDS politics in search of calmer seas.

CHALLENGES TO AIDS ACTIVISM

As the AIDS crisis enters its second decade, the biggest challenge to activists comes from this backlash from society, researchers, drug companies, and advocates for patients with other diseases.[32] But there are other challenges as well, products of the unique history and culture of the activist movement itself.

First, the movement and the epidemic are becoming increasingly diverse. When ACT UP was founded in 1987, homosexual men (most of them white) constituted 70 percent of Americans with AIDS and the vast majority of AIDS activists. Today, such men make up 55 percent of people with AIDS, and the percentage is shrinking.[33] The increasing numbers of drug users, people of color, and women at risk for HIV infection are greatly concerned about preventing the spread of HIV. This means that the strategies that were so effective in the gay community must be reevaluated and adapted to the particular cultures, languages, and institutions of the communities newly at risk.

Moreover, these communities are besieged with other overwhelming social maladies, many of them linked to the HIV epidemic. Effective AIDS strategies for these groups must address issues of poverty, racism, violence, drug abuse, teenage pregnancy, abortion, and access to health care—issues that were less important to the earlier gay, white AIDS activists.

A second type of diversity that divides the activist movement relates to the serologic status and agenda of the participants. The early activists were generally HIV–positive or had full-blown AIDS, which accounted for their devotion to the quest for effective drugs. Attracted by the success and high visibility of the activists, recent entrants into the AIDS movement, some of them seronegative, have more complex motivations. The primary goal of these people is often to eradicate the social ills of homophobia, racism, and sexism. The conflict between the "treatment" activists and the "social agenda" activists has led to infighting within the movement and even to the breakup of ACT UP into two distinct chapters in San Francisco.[34]

The activist movement has also been wrenched by disagreement over strategy. As would be expected of a movement whose tactics range from disrupting the New York Stock Exchange to publishing position papers that evaluate new reverse transcriptase inhibitors, activists disagree on whether confrontation or collaboration is the most effective strategy. Those primarily concerned with treatment have generally favored working with the system, because it is the biomedical establishment that must be counted on to develop, test, and approve new drugs. More radical factions argue for a more confrontational strategy.[35] Larry Kramer called for riots at the Sixth International Conference on AIDS.[36] Although this call was promptly repudiated by other activists,[4] the fact that it was made by ACT UP's founder exposed the wide range of opinions on strategy within the movement.

Perhaps the greatest challenge to AIDS activism is posed by the merciless nature of the disease itself. Although activists have succeeded in demanding that the world take note of the urgency of the epidemic, that very urgency is what robs the movement daily of its best soldiers through burnout, illness, and death . . . .

REFERENCES

1. Strickland SP. Medical research: public policy and power politics. In: Cater D, Lee PR, eds. Politics in health. Huntington, N.Y.: Robert E. Kneger Publishing, 1979:75–97.
2. Hamilton PA. Health care consumerism. St. Louis: C. V. Mosby, 1982.
3. Bennett JT. Health research charities: image and reality. Washington, D.C.: Capital Research Center, 1990.
4. Wachter, RM. The fragile coalition: scientists, activists, and AIDS. New York: St. Martin's Press, 1991.

5. Leo J. When activism becomes gangsterism. U.S. News & World Report. February 5, 1990:18.
6. Dowd M. Bush chides protesters on 'excesses.' New York Times. August 17, 1991:7.
7. Angell M. A dual approach to the AIDS epidemic. N Engl J Med 1991;324:1498–500.
8. Bayer R. Public health policy and the AIDS epidemic—an end to HIV exceptionalism? N Engl J Med 1991;324:1500–4.
9. Shilts R. And the band played on: politics, people, and the AIDS epidemic. New York: St. Martin's Press, 1987.
10. Bayer R. Private acts, social consequences: AIDS and the politics of public health. New Brunswick, N.J.: Rutgers University Press, 1991.
11. Kramer L. Reports from the holocaust: the making of an AIDS activist. New York: St. Martin's Press, 1989.
12. Salholz E. The future of gay America. Newsweek, March 12, 1990:20–5.
13. Masterson-Allen S, Brown P. Public reaction to toxic waste contamination: analysis of a social movement. Int J Health Serv 1990;20:485–500.
14. Kolata G. U. S. to expand use of AIDS medicines. New York Times. May 19, 1990:A8.
15. Chase M. Burroughs-Wellcome cuts price of AZT under pressure from AIDS activists. Wall Street Journal. September 19, 1989:A3.
16. Little M (Malcolm X). By any means necessary. New York: Pathfinder Press, 1970.
17. Blumberg RL. Civil rights: the 1960s freedom struggle. Boston: Twayne, 1984.
18. Colaiaco JA. Martin Luther King, Jr.: apostle of militant nonviolence. New York: St. Martin's Press, 1988.
19. Grossman H. Keep politics out of scientific research. New York Times. August 19, 1990;III:13.
20. Thompson D. The AIDS political machine. Time. January 22, 1990:1–5.
21. Krauthammer C. AIDS: getting more than its share? Time. June 25, 1990:80.
22. Winkenwerder W, Kessler AR, Stolec RM. Federal spending for illness caused by the human immunodeficiency virus. N Engl J Med 1989; 320:1598–603.
23. McIntosh H. AIDS lobby earns respect from cancer leaders. J Natl Cancer Inst 1990;82:730–2.
24. Fuchs VR. Who shall live? Health, economics, and social choice. New York: Basic Books, 1974.
25. Delaney M. The case for patient access to experimental therapy. J Infect Dis 1989;159:416–9.
26. Kolata G. Unorthodox trials of AIDS drugs are allowed by FDA to go on. New York Times. March 9, 1990:A1.
27. Public Health Service, HHS. Expanded availability of investigational new drugs through a parallel track mechanism for people with AIDS and HIV-related disease. Fed Regist 1990;55:20856–60.
28. Annas GJ. Faith (healing), hope and charity at the FDA: the politics of AIDS drug trials. Villanova Law Rev 1989:34:771–97.
29. Stall R, Ekstrand M, Pollack L, McKusick L, Coates TJ. Relapse from safer sex: the next challenge for AIDS prevention efforts. J Acquir Immune Defic Syndr 1990;3:1181–7.
30. Vollmer T. How far with the politics of anger? San Francisco Sentinel. June 28, 1990:9.
31. *Idem.* Three points for ACT-UP to consider. San Francisco Sentinel. August 2, 1990:9.
32. Garrison J. The AIDS research backlash. San Francisco Examiner. December 17, 1989:A1.
33. Update: acquired immunodeficiency syndrome—United States, 1981–1990. MMWR 1991; 40:358–69.

34. Kneger LM. Ideology clash underlies split within ACT UP. San Francisco Examiner. October 14, 1990:B1.
35. Spiers HR. AIDS and civil disobedience. Hastings Cent Rep 1989; 19(6):34–5.
36. Kramer L. A call to riot. Outweek Magazine. March 14, 1990:36–8.

4

Green Monkeys and Dark Continents: AIDS and Racism

Tamsin Wilton

Although there is a general recognition among more thoughtful people that categorizing AIDS as the 'gay plague' is both wrong and offensive, there is still a widely held belief in something equally suspect called 'African AIDS'. Many who consider themselves well informed still subscribe to the (discredited) belief that HIV/AIDS came from Africa. This outmoded belief is often accompanied by a whole set of wildly inaccurate generalizations about the 'epidemic in Africa'. . . . Where do such ideas originate, and why are they still so widely held to be true?

One favorite theory (among white commentators) of the origins of HIV/AIDS goes as follows: HIV is a mutation of a similar virus which is found in African green monkeys and was somehow passed on to humans. It was taken to Haiti by migrant Black workers, who infected a 'pool' of Haitian male prostitutes, who then infected US gay men vacationing in Haiti. The US gay men, the story continues, because of their sexual promiscuity and ready access to international travel, sparked off the epidemic in the first world. Although this theory was based on very flimsy evidence, and has since been rejected by some of the scientists who originally suggested it, it achieved instant popularity with the press and media and received widespread publicity. Maps showing the putative global route taken by the epidemic as dramatic arrows radiating from the heart of Africa became com-

"Green Monkeys and Dark Continents: AIDS and Racism" by Tamsin Wilton, from *Antibody Politic: AIDS and Society* (Cheltenham, UK: New Clarion Press, 1992), pp. 75–93. Copyright © 1992 by New Clarion Press.

monplace in books, magazines, newspapers and television documentaries. So what truth is there in the theory that HIV originated in Africa? Probably none.

As Haringey Council's Race Equality Unit records, in its paper *AIDS and Racism*, sophisticated genetic tests have now indicated that the virus which infects green monkeys is fundamentally different to HIV, so different as to discredit claims that one is a mutation of the other. Epidemiological studies, meanwhile, have led researchers to conclude that there is no evidence to suggest that the virus was present in Africa at an earlier time than in the United States. Dr Richard Tedder, a virologist at the Middlesex Hospital, states, 'I find no evidence of this being an archival virus in Africa. Prevalence rates in the African continent started to go up at about the same time as they did in America and Europe.' HIV, in other words, is as recent an arrival in Africa as it is elsewhere in the world. Indeed, some commentators suggest that there is just as much evidence to suggest that the virus was 'exported' from the USA to Africa in supplies of blood and blood products. Although I am emphatically *not* suggesting that this is the case, it is clearly important to recognize that while one of these competing explanations has been widely publicized (and the African origins story is consequently a familiar one to most people in Britain), the other has not.

There is no consensus among the scientific community about the geographical origins of HIV, and the green monkey hypothesis has been resoundingly disproved, yet although many British newspapers, books and television news broadcasts and documentaries have published detailed accounts of this nasty little fiction, there has been a noticeable lack of public correction or retraction. Only one television documentary, *Monkey Business*, broadcast late at night on Channel 4 in 1989, offered a detailed rejection of the green monkey hypothesis—only to replace it with the suggestion that the CIA were responsible for developing HIV in their germ warfare laboratories. Why is something as tenuous as the association between Africa and AIDS met with such wholesale credulity?

THE WHITE MAN'S GRAVE

The positioning of Africa in Western accounts of the epidemic can only be understood in the historical context of colonialism, slavery and social Darwinism. The white nations who invaded the African continent, who set about systematically destroying local culture and the local economy, who set in motion the shameful barbarity of the slave trade and who later imposed the grossly inappropriate values and structures of Victorian capitalism on the people whose world they had done their best to destroy, were obliged to justify their actions to themselves and the folks back home. If Africans were recognized as human beings, with a civilization, religious beliefs and 'high' feelings, the wholesale destruction wreaked upon them would be exposed for the bar-

barism which it in fact was. So the politically and socially expedient notion of the 'savage', a creature lower down the evolutionary ladder than 'civilized' white people, was deployed, and Africa was labeled the Dark Continent, an embodiment of all that was untamed, wild, uncontrollable, bestial and dangerous. Additionally, the early colonists, ill prepared for the climate and environment of Africa, and unprotected by natural immunity or medical prophylaxis, sickened and died in great numbers from unfamiliar diseases.

For whites growing up in Britain in the first half of the twentieth century, the familiar image of Africa and Africans was an uncompromising legacy from the ideology of colonialism. Africa was represented as a huge, hot, undifferentiated and oppressive chaos, which dedicated and masterful white people were struggling to bring under the yoke of civilization. It was swarming with flies, dirt and horrific diseases, and its people were ignorant savages who worshiped idols, let their babies die and killed the missionaries and doctors who tried to help them. Men like Albert Schweitzer and Dr. Livingstone, together with the swarms of missionaries sent out to bring the pitiful savage under the rule of God, were the heroes of Africa. There was a strong thread of uncontrolled sexuality running through these accounts, reflecting the British dread of sex. Africans did not wear clothes and they did not know that you had to be married in order to have sex; African men had huge penises, and were likely to offer a white man a cow in exchange for a white woman to add to their collection of wives.

It is tempting to see this ridiculous and insulting picture as an outmoded leftover, something as archaic as whalebone stays, and as risible. But such vigorously promoted fictions do not simply relinquish their hold on the mind when exposed to the cold light of reality, as the ready welcome offered to the 'African origins of AIDS' fiction indicates. Such an account, devoid of rigorous scientific proof, is only credible in the context of the archaic and racist fictions of colonialism. It is only comprehensible to the racist imagination. Thus the findings in one of the London hospitals early in 1992, showing that a high percentage of pregnant women testing positive for HIV antibodies during a screening program had connections with Africa, were given copious press coverage. The voice of reason, cautioning that generalizations could not and should not be drawn from one survey undertaken in one hospital (and pointing out that, after all, an even greater percentage of the women sampled had connections with London and had had heterosexual sex!), had little chance of being heard over the determination to justify the familiar narrative of racism.

MONKEYING AROUND

The idea that a virus could be passed from monkeys to Black Africans (nobody had ever suggested that white Africans were involved) implies either a clear biological similarity between Black Africans and monkeys, or some vaguely disgusting kind of contact between them. Indeed, *Africa Report* (November/December 1988) records that the South African media, under apartheid, published claims that AIDS was due to ritual and sexual contact between Black Africans and baboons. Such outlandish suggestions find ready agreement in the racist imagination. Research carried out by Jenny Kitzinger and David Miller in 1991 shows that people from all walks of life believe that Africans have sex with animals, including bulls, gorillas and monkeys. Some of their interviewees went further, blaming 'Pakis' having sex with gorillas or monkeys for 'bringing it [AIDS] here'.

Such statements reveal non-white cultures to be an imaginary world constructed, as it were, from the 'missing bits' of white culture, almost a looking-glass reversal where anything might happen. This is hardly surprising, given that people are obliged to fall back on their imagination to construct for them a workable mental model of anything about which they do not have ready access to alternative sources of information. Television is overwhelmingly the most powerful (and credible) source of information in most people's lives. It is certainly cited by most British people as their major source of information about AIDS. Yet British television offers us a picture of Africa which is both limited and distorted. We are obliged to flesh out the bones of an Africa culturally constructed from Tarzan films, wildlife documentaries, brief film clips from television news items about famine, civil war or disaster, and compassion-a-thons such as Live Aid and Comic Relief. With precious little information to balance the scenes of famine, drought and nomadic despair, it is perhaps not surprising that otherwise intelligent people in Britain find it hard to believe the truth that not all Africans live in mud huts in jungles positively teeming with monkeys, that actually the majority seldom see a monkey.

In fact, the pattern of the epidemic in Africa is not quite as different from that in Europe and the USA as we would like to believe. It is not true, for example, that HIV is most prevalent in rural areas (where monkeys are common); rather, HIV infection and AIDS are most often found in towns and cities, as is the case in the UK. Yet, to judge by media representations in the UK, there *is* no urban Africa. It is perhaps salutary to recognize that many Africans are much more aware of the realities of the relationship between Africa and the (over)developed nations than most people in Europe. In some African countries, the local dialect word for AIDS is the same as that for foreign aid.

The same racist imagination paints a lurid and inaccurate picture of the epidemic in Africa, to such a degree that many people believe that 'AIDS is rife' throughout the continent, that whole populations are dying, and that widespread sexual promiscuity combined with peculiar sexual practices is to blame. In fact, of course Africa is not one country, with one epidemic. Rather, it is made up of many nations with many differing rates and patterns of spread, exactly like Europe. How many British people would be happy for Romania to be taken as the best example of what happens in Europe? Different nations in the African continent may have barely comparable standards of living, economic structures, languages, health care systems or social mores, and it is simply not true that they share one epidemic. Reported cases of AIDS across the 53 African countries vary from 0.3 per million in Nigeria to 568 per million in Congo, with a handful of countries where no cases have been reported at all. The average rate of AIDS cases taken over Africa as a whole is around 78.1 per million, compared to an average taken across the United States of 464 per million, a figure which equals that of Uganda. There are only four countries in Africa which have reported numbers of AIDS cases as bad as, or worse than, the USA. In comparison, the United Kingdom reports 48 cases of AIDS per million, Ireland 31, France 145 and Spain 158. The WHO estimates that half of the global total of 283,010 cases of AIDS are in the United States, a quarter in sub–Saharan Africa and 14 per cent in Europe (figures taken from reports to the World Health Organization by 1 September 1990).

There are reasons to be cautious about such figures, of course. Crucially, they represent the number of cases of AIDS in a country, not the numbers of people with HIV. It is not possible to state categorically how many cases of HIV infection we may expect for every diagnosed case of AIDS, and estimates vary widely. However, it is probably a cautious estimate to suggest that there may be ten people with HIV for every one person diagnosed with AIDS. On the basis of the best figures available, the WHO estimates (1991) that there are a million HIV+ people in North America, a further million in Latin America, close to half a million in Africa and five hundred thousand in Europe. This implies that the situation in Uganda (or the USA), with a likely rate of infection of 4,640 per million, is certainly very grave. Additionally, the number of cases reported is almost certainly an underestimate in most countries, for a variety of reasons. In a wealthy country like Britain, AIDS may go undiagnosed because the patient does not fall into one of the misleading 'risk groups', or may go unreported in an attempt to avoid social stigma. In a very poor country, where the annual health care budget per head of population may be as low as £4–£5, diagnostic technology may not be widely available, many people may simply live too far away from medical centers to get help, local healing traditions may take precedence over Western medicine, or an individual may not be able to take time off from the essentials of subsistence living to seek medical attention. Additionally, people already living at the limit of their physical strength, their health taxed by overwork, malnutrition and frequent exposure to infections and parasites. are likely to become ill and to die very rapidly, before there is time to start the often complex practicalities of consulting a doctor.

On the other hand, some experts have claimed that the situation in many African countries may have been exaggerated. Malaria, for example, frequently gives a false positive result on an HIV antibody test, as do certain other infections and conditions. Testing to eliminate all such possibilities is not feasible when operating under the constraints of poorly resourced and understaffed health services.

Whether the figures are accurate or not, it is clear that the progress of the epidemic is not comparable across all African countries, any more than across all European countries. Nevertheless, it is obvious that someone who becomes infected with HIV in a poor country in central Africa, or in one of the areas where civil wars are being fought, has a very different outlook from someone in a wealthy family in central London. The numbers may not be as high as they are in the United States, but the implications of AIDS for some African nations are nevertheless devastating.

THE HEALTH CONSEQUENCES OF COLONIALISM

This is not the place to detail the complex outline of the impact of colonialism on African countries. Other writers have identified the many negative consequences which colonial exploitation has had for the health of Black Africans. Far from being the Black people's savior from disease, the white invaders in fact disrupted complex strategies developed over centuries by indigenous peoples to prevent diseases such as sleeping sickness from taking hold. They also introduced new and previously unknown diseases (such as syphilis), and the migrant labor schemes they imposed brought malnutrition and general immiseration to the populations they controlled. The contemporary picture is no better. Black workers in white-owned mines have high rates of respiratory infections, or are vulnerable to the toxic effects of substances such as uranium, while entire nations which have been coerced into replacing agricultural self-sufficiency with cash-crop farming (producing luxury goods such as coffee for the European market) find their economies disastrously tied to the vagaries of world markets and multinational corporations, while their agricultural production is obliged to wrestle with all the problems associated with monoculture, such as pest control and soil exhaustion.

It is against this background that the impact of AIDS on Africa must be seen. If you are lucky enough to live in one of the wealthier African countries, whose cities are large and cosmopolitan, and if you are lucky enough to have a well-paid job and a good education, you will have access to health care as good as any in the North, and your general health is likely to be as good as, or better than, that of someone in a similar position in Paris, Madrid or London. If you were to contract HIV, sophisticated diagnostic and therapeutic support would be available to you.

If you are unlucky enough to live in a rural subsistence community in one of the poorer countries, the story is very different. In such countries, there are not enough trained doctors to go round, the most basic medical necessities are in short supply, and essentials that are taken for granted in Britain, like clean drinking water. fresh foods or even soap, are hard to come by. Testing equipment needed to diagnose HIV is costly, and must be bought at the expense of other, perhaps more urgently needed equipment. To provide new, sterile syringes and needles for every injection or blood test for every patient (a procedure taken for granted in British clinics and hospitals) would eat up most of the annual health care budget, so injecting equipment must perforce be re-used. The drugs used to postpone deterioration of the immune system in people with HIV, or to combat the various opportunistic infections associated with AIDS, are very costly, and might just as well be on Mars as far as most third world countries are concerned. Uganda, for example, one of the worst affected countries, had in 1988 an annual AIDS budget of less than $5 million. AZT, the drug most widely used in the USA to prolong the life of people with HIV/AIDS, cost in 1988 $10,000 per patient per year. This stark economic equation holds true, of course, for any eventual cure or vaccine which may be developed. In other words, it is not the 'promiscuity' or strange sexual practices of Darkest Africa which have resulted in the rapid spread of HIV in some African countries; it is poverty.

It is important to stress this, because experience has shown that many white British people who should know better hold very bizarre views about the sexual behavior of Black Africans. A Radio 4 phone-in host was the center of a small storm in 1991 when he hung up in disgust on a (male) caller who said, *vis-à-vis* Black Africans and AIDS, 'Well, we just don't know what goes on in those mud huts, do we?' It is tempting to write such blatant nonsense off as the thoughtless prejudice of an ill-educated few, but such views (albeit less crudely expressed) have been aired in surprising places. Thus in *AIDS*, a textbook about HIV/AIDS for younger schoolchildren by Alison and David Kilpatrick, we find the statement that: 'In central Africa, heterosexual men are generally more promiscuous than in Europe and America, and going to a prostitute is more socially acceptable. It seems likely that prostitutes in particular, and promiscuous behavior generally, have made central Africa the most AIDS–ridden area in the world.' (The same book tells us that the only reason lesbians are a 'low risk group' is that they are seldom promiscuous. This husband-and-wife team clearly has a moral message to promote!)

It is clear that, while such unsubstantiated and offensive rubbish is being taught in our schools, health promotion which aims to equip everyone with the knowledge and motivation to protect themselves from HIV infection is fighting a losing battle. Just as homophobia is proving lethal to heterosexuals in the context of HIV/AIDS, so racism is proving potentially lethal to those whose prejudice and bigotry overrules logic and understanding.

RACISM AND AIDS IN BRITAIN

Overt racism has touched almost every aspect of the British response to the epidemic. This is seen most clearly in the enthusiastic acceptance of the African origins story, and in subsequent health promotion efforts. Thus, in

1987 the Terrence Higgins Trust produced an informative booklet, *AIDS and HIV: Medical Briefing*, which listed, under the heading 'Who can get HIV infection?', 'People having sex with people who have lived in or visited central Africa', commenting that 'anyone who has lived there or visited the area and had sexual intercourse there could . . . be at risk'. There was no mention of the potential risks of visiting certain cities in the United States and having sexual intercourse there, despite the fact that, statistically, the likelihood of becoming infected with HIV while visiting some US cities was much greater than in some central African countries! (THT subsequently apologized for this, after a Black woman pointed it out publicly at a conference.) Similarly, the blood transfusion service publicly advise that 'Men and women who have had sex at any time since 1977 with men or women living in African countries, except those on the Mediterranean . . . must *not* give blood.' It does not take long for a supposed risk attached to those who have had sex with Africans to be expanded within the racist imagination to include all people with a black skin. Thus, the medical correspondent of *The Times*, Dr. Stuttard, publicly labeled young Afro-Caribbean men *living in Britain* as a high risk group in the spread of HIV, an illogical statement based on absolutely no scientific evidence whatsoever, and clearly racist.

The effect on white people of believing that HIV/AIDS is something which is more likely to affect Black people is dangerous in the same way as the belief among some heterosexuals that HIV only affects gays. It is a relief to be able to believe that AIDS is just one more disaster taking place in distant Africa, familiar stage for disease and death. Once the association has been created between blackness and HIV, white people are less likely to see themselves as at risk, and less likely to take steps to protect themselves. Additionally, blackness is seen as intrinsically contaminating within the colonialist logic of racism, in much the same way as homosexuality is seen as intrinsically contaminating within the logic of heterosexism, or female prostitution (and female sexuality generally) as intrinsically contaminating within the logic of sexism. Black people have long been associated in the white racist imagination with animality, perverse and insatiable sexuality and feckless irresponsibility. With a sigh of relief, the chaste white onlooker is now able to imagine HIV as the logical consequence of such behavior, so different from that of our own dear queen and all her subjects. Once 'risk' has been ascribed to a group so demonstrably alien, a now-familiar warped logic demands that those identified as 'at risk' become perceived as posing a risk to others. So, assured on all sides that Black people are at risk for HIV/AIDS, white people are less likely to protect themselves against HIV, or to call for steps to be taken to support and protect the Blacks they believe to be at risk, and more likely to attempt to protect themselves from *the risk to their own health* which they believe Black people to represent.

The implications of the racist response to HIV/AIDS are, therefore, far more dangerous to Black people than to white people. Indeed, reports from many countries indicate that Black people have been subjected to abuse, increased discrimination and even violence related to the belief that they are in some way responsible for AIDS. Thus, African students at Hangzhou University in China were harassed and isolated by their colleagues as a result of the conviction that contact with Black Africans could transmit HIV; Belgian parliamentary spokesman Paul van Stallen proclaimed that 'We shouldn't pay others to come here and be a danger for our own people', as Belgium decided to test African students for HIV; and all African students at one Russian medical school were compulsorily tested (examples taken from *The Third Epidemic*). In Britain, the National Front have distributed a leaflet, entitled 'Conspiracy to Destroy our Nation through AIDS', which asserts that 'AIDS–infested Africans are brought into Britain from AIDS–infested Africa . . . to live on the dole and social security etc. (at our expense).'

Racism takes its toll on the mental and physical health of all people of color living in white society, and HIV once again may be fitted into a pre-existing picture of oppression and disadvantage.

CONCLUSION

Racism, along with all the other 'isms' acts to spend the progress of the epidemic, not to halt it. It impedes the process of recognizing that all are at risk, thereby putting dangerous obstacles in the way of health education. The legacy of racist colonialist exploitation acts to hasten the progress of the virus across the poor countries in central Africa, while ensuring that the valuable lesson to be learned from the pattern of transmission in these countries remains lost on the policy makers of the developed world, who distance themselves from what their racism tells them is a 'Black problem', caused by promiscuity and backwardness. The inequitable distribution of the world's resources means that HIV hits hardest at those people to whom the most basic necessities of life are already denied. Such people are disproportionately Black, a pattern which is not confined to the economic inequalities maintained between the (over)developed nations and the third world, but is repeated in microcosm in the inner cities of the first world. It is structural and institutional racism, not innate savagery, which increases the risk of HIV infection for peoples of color.

As always, HIV cannot be seen as a new problem. It fits into the familiar and shameful narratives of racism, so that poor Black and Latino people in the USA have disproportionately high rates of HIV infection, as they have disproportionately high rates of TB; so that Afro-Caribbean people from China to Britain have 'AIDS carrier' shouted at them along with all the other abuse; so that information is not made available to those whose cultural and religious beliefs make them 'difficult' for white people to approach; so that lesbians and gay men of color are seldom recognized as in need of support; so that official bodies such as the blood transfusion service encourage racism by refusing blood contaminated by association with Africa; so that Black groups find it hard to get essential funding; so that white groups see racism as a 'separate issue'. A separate issue is, of course, just what it is *not*. Dr. Jonathan Mann, when he was director of the World Health Organization, was clear that prejudice and discrimination, in all their forms, represented the 'third epidemic'; that the health and safety of us all depend upon the recognition that bigotry, whether directed at Blacks, gays, drug users or those already infected, is the single greatest threat to our ability to defeat AIDS.

PART TWO

Public Policy and AIDS

5

Myths and Illusions: The Media and AIDS Policy

Stella Z. Theodoulou, Gloria Y. Guevara, and Henrik Minnassians

Acquired immunodeficiency syndrome (AIDS) was first acknowledged in the United States in 1981 and since then, AIDS has had an unprecedented effect upon society.[1] Few other diseases in this century have had such an impact and been greeted with such hostility and fear. In the United States and the rest of the world, the mass media has played a central role in constructing individuals' knowledge and attitudes towards AIDS. Indeed, Street (1988) argues that AIDS may be the first media disease. Critics of media AIDS coverage argue that, in the majority of the mass media coverage, AIDS has been treated as a condition that effects marginalized groups such as homosexuals, intravenous drug users, and those who engage in promiscuous behavior. Yet in later coverage AIDS has been presented to the public as a disease that can threaten everyone and anyone; a truly nondiscriminating virus. These two seemingly different interpretations can be found in the way the medical scientific community has also classified the epidemic and in turn how American policymakers have responded to the demands of the virus (Theodoulou, 1996). For instance, the early designation by the medical community of AIDS was gay-related immune deficiency syndrome (GRID) and the mass media responded by proclaiming a "gay plague" was sweeping the world. Much of the coverage of GRID was that it was a disease that had somehow grown out of or was the natural expression of the "disease" of homosexuality itself (Boffin & Gupta, 1990). Those inflicted with AIDS were depicted as being gay men who had several sex partners and whose sexuality and sexual practices were so "abnormal" as to be responsible for their own physical demise. A picture of gay life emerged in the media that was basically and irrevocably at odds with accepted American lifestyles (Feldman & Johnson, 1986).

In this study we examine how the American mass media, represented by six of the nation's largest and most respected daily newspapers, has managed to handle the reporting of the epidemic. How do the media messages about AIDS change over time? Do the media cover, in a responsible manner, public health concerns of contagion, plague, and death? Has there been any change in the amount and extent of coverage? All of these questions are examined through a longitudinal content analysis of *The New York Times, Los Angeles Times, Wall Street Journal, Chicago Tribune, Washington Post,* and *San Francisco Chronicle.* The time period under examination is January 1981 to July 1994.

The reasons for this study are, like many empirical undertakings, numerous, but for the most part the study was motivated by two concerns. First, has media coverage in any way affected the policymaking response? In short, the first reason for this analysis was to examine the relationship between the media agenda and the policy agenda. The second reason for the analysis was stimulated by the conclusion drawn at the Freedom Forum's Unity 1994 Conference.[2] The general consensus of American reporters covering AIDS issues was that stories about the disease are fast disappearing from the news pages, despite the continuing growth in numbers of people infected. In many cases, editors contend that the issue has been covered sufficiently, and that there is nothing new to report. As Jesse Mangaliman of the *New York Newsday* stated, "I think the biggest challenge in selling the story to your editors is constantly and everyday reeducating them and making them aware of what the issue is, even if you have to do AIDS 101. You have to work harder when you're selling an AIDS story, because it's been around for so long, editors will tell you they are tired of hearing it" (Mangaliman, 1994, p. 2). Through an examination of newspaper coverage this study attempts to see whether the reporters' assertions are true.

The analysis begins with a review of the existing literature on news media coverage of AIDS and then proceeds to a discussion of the six newspapers' coverage of the epidemic from 1981 to 1994. While the focus of the analysis is on coverage in the American newspapers, reference will be made to broad trends that have affected the Western world as a whole.

AIDS IN THE NEWS MEDIA

In the last fourteen years, AIDS has commanded an enormous amount of media interest. In 1985, United Press International reported that AIDS was one of the top four newsmaking issues. In the same year, the Associated Press and the Encyclopaedia Britannica ranked the AIDS issue as the fifth and sixth, respectively, most-reported issue on a worldwide basis. Hughey, Norton, and

Sullivan-Norton (1989, pp. 56–57) state that these same services all ranked AIDS ninth in international news value in 1986. Such coverage cannot help but to have affected the way society as a whole looks at and understands the ramifications of the epidemic.

A large number of the qualitative studies that have been conducted constantly refer to the media as an important, if not crucial, source of AIDS information (Bray & Chapman, 1991; Ross, 1989; Crimp, 1992; Ross & Carson, 1988; Dolan, Corber & Zacow, 1990; Carducci, Frasca, Matteelli et al., 1990). Another large group of studies has acknowledged the significant impact that the media has had on individual, mass, and governmental attitudes and belief systems (White, Phillips, Pitt et al., 1988; Abraham, Sheeran, Abrams, et al., 1991; Tulloch, 1989 & 1992; Kitzinger, 1990; Kitzinger & Miller, 1991).

Much of the research on media coverage of AIDS concentrates on the American news media (Albert, 1986a & 1986b; Baker, 1986; Hughey, Norton & Sullivan-Norton, 1989; King, 1990; Austin, 1990; Clarke, 1991 & 1992; Nelkin, 1991; Rogers, Dearing & Chang, 1991; Colby & Cook, 1991) and the British media (Wellings, 1988; Murray, 1991; Beharrell, 1991 & 1993; Berridge, 1991). However, the news media in Australia (Lupton, 1994; Penny, 1988; French, 1986), France (Herzlich & Pierret, 1989), Puerto Rico (Cunningham, 1989), West Germany (Jones, 1992), and Canada (Clarke, 1991) have also been analyzed.

On reading these studies, it can be concluded that there are several broad patterns of AIDS reporting. In all countries, authors conclude that there appear to be phases or peaks in coverage. The numbers vary from nation to nation, but pivotal dates are shared; for example, four phases in France (Herzlich & Pierret, 1989) and three peaks in the United States (Rogers, Dearing & Chang, 1991). According to the above literature, there are also changes that all nations share in the focus of the coverage over time. The pattern seems to be one of stigmatization—concern with civil rights violations—and heterosexualization of the virus. Several of the studies have found there to be a symbiotic relationship between media coverage and government policy about AIDS. For example, Cunningham (1989) argues that, in Puerto Rico, press coverage was used as a means of contrasting the ideologies of political leaders rather then communicating information about AIDS to the general public. Thus, Cunningham concludes that the general perception in Puerto Rico is that AIDS is a political, rather than a medical, question. In the United Kingdom, government policy has often been contradicted by information conveyed in media coverage (Wellings, 1988). While in the United States, the general neglect and lack of political leadership on the AIDS question (Theodoulou, 1996) is reflected by the contradictory and confusing coverage of the issue by the media (Nelkin, 1991).

AMERICAN MEDIA COVERAGE

The American media in the case of AIDS has constructed a social reality for societal understanding of the epidemic. Early AIDS reporting in the United States created the foundations for the myths that have stigmatized certain groups based on their lifestyle choices (Hughey, Norton & Sullivan-Norton, 1989). From its discovery in 1981 until the early 1990s AIDS has been reported in this manner.

The American media's early coverage from 1981 to 1983 set the stage for how AIDS was to be understood by society: it was a disease that primarily affected gay men, Haitians, and "others." During this period AIDS was introduced into society by the media as a disease of "others," one that has been perceived by society as a result of individual lifestyle choices rather than as resulting from circumstances beyond an individual's control. People inflicted with the "gay plague" were portrayed by the media as experiencing a reign of terror, a death sentence, justified by an exponentially increasing death toll, throwing the gay community into panic (Feldman & Johnson, 1986). Early reporting of AIDS dealt primarily with the groups afflicted and it was in this context that AIDS was labeled by the media as a disease afflicting those individuals who participated in "high risk" behavior; behavior that existed outside mainstream America. The sexual conservatism of the media reflects its efforts to avoid alienating its broad readership (Nelkin, 1991).

In 1983, the media's coverage of AIDS peaked with the publication of Dr. Anthony Fauci's May 6th article in the Journal of the American Medical Association (JAMA). Fauci, director of the National Institute of Allergy and Infectious Disease, raised the possibility that AIDS may be transmitted to the entire population by "routine close contact" with infected individuals (Nelkin, 1991). Such an announcement implied to the general population that everyone was at risk. At the same time, the media carried reports of heterosexual cases of infection; such reports created panic and hysteria among the public. AIDS as a homosexual disease received little media coverage, but AIDS as a disease from which everyone was at risk was more newsworthy. Of course, Fauci's hypothesis of contagion through casual contact was incorrect, and after reassurance from the scientific community of this fact, media coverage of AIDS declined by the end of the summer of 1983 (Nelkin, 1991). Around this same period, the emergence of "high risk" groups begins to take a more concrete form. This phenomenon helped the scientific community to reassure the public through the media that as long as they did not engage in "risky" behavior they would be safe from being infected with AIDS.

The 1980s was a period in which the scientific community was slowly discovering more about the disease of AIDS. However, the attention given to AIDS by the media steadily declined until 1985. In 1985, as in 1983, coverage increased due to an unexpected announcement: the movie star Rock Hudson had AIDS. During this time period, Hudson's illness was not the only phenomenon that was able to attract the media's attention. There was also the emergence of Ryan White, a young hemophiliac who was infected with AIDS from a blood transfusion. These two announcements raised several issues regarding AIDS in the media discussion. The first questioned the safety of the national blood supply; if an innocent child such as Ryan White could receive "tainted" blood, could the general public be at risk too? A second issue raised by the media in their discussion was the need to develop an accurate HIV antibody test; not just for the general population, but also for screening of the blood supply. Another question raised in the media by the White case concerned the way children infected with AIDS should be treated by society. In spite of the intensity of such issues, media coverage declined after 1985 and did not peak again until 1987. It was now the media's task to inform the public without creating a panic among them.

The events of 1985 further reinforced and perpetuated the myths and stereotypes surrounding AIDS. For the most part, AIDS, as perceived by society and as reflected in the media, is a result of an individual exercising their own lifestyle choices, as opposed to succumbing to uncontrollable external forces. This concept is in no way limited to the homosexual identity with AIDS. Adams (1989) argues this is true of all groups associated with AIDS. He refers to this as the "Five H's" which include: hemophiliacs, homosexuals, Haitians, heroin addicts, and hookers. With the exception of hemophiliacs, the other four groups are viewed as being responsible for their own illness because of their perceived deviancy. Infected individuals are viewed as playing a role in their own demise, their situation being the result of lifestyle choices that could have been avoided with behavior modification. Hemophiliacs, in contrast, do not carry the same burden as the other four groups; their situation is perceived as the result of misfortune due to receiving "tainted" blood. Their situation is depicted by the news media as an accident—while homosexuals and IV drug users could adjust their behavior to avoid exposure, hemophiliacs could not. These lifestyle images as conveyed by the media affect an individual's moral construction of AIDS. Thus, the media presented the general public with the notion of "high risk groups" and "innocent victims." Therefore, the relevance of the construction of the AIDS "victim" by the media so early in the course of the epidemic is that it has set the foundation for how society views AIDS. It is still very much a disease of "others."

Since 1985, AIDS has also been used as a weapon by groups whose agenda has been to punish what they view as abnormal and immoral. For example, since Rock Hudson's death, members of the religious right have repeatedly used AIDS to proclaim that the disease is God's way of showing displeasure with the homosexual lifestyle. To such individuals, AIDS was not only a known danger, but also an expression of divine will (Hughey, Norton & Sullivan-Norton, 1989). During this period, the morality and lifestyle argument received considerable media attention. The disease of "others" was now being used by groups to target immoral behavior, such as premarital sex, homosexuality, illegal drug use, and prostitution, that the Moral Majority suggested God was punishing. After 1985, the reporting of AIDS, for the most part, can be viewed in the context of risk reporting. News stories can be seen to either depict certain lifestyle characteristics associated with the disease or to relay information from the scientific community. Thus, AIDS was being used in many ways by the media. For example, AIDS stories were used to generate information about other life dangers and other diseases, to teach moral lessons and explain lifestyle choices, to illuminate social and economic problems, and finally, AIDS stories were used as both a defensive and offensive weapon (Hughey, Norton, & Sullivan-Norton, 1989, p. 66).

In 1987, media coverage once again peaked (Rogers, Dearing, & Chang, 1991), this time attributed to public federal government recommendations on testing and screening procedures and President Reagan's first formal acknowledgment of AIDS. It was at this point in time that authors such as Colby and Cook (1991) argue that the policy agenda was affected. From 1981 to 1987 the Reagan administration completely ignored AIDS as an epidemic (Theodoulou, 1996); this lack of acknowledgment is reflected in the media's inconsistent coverage of AIDS from 1981 (Colby & Cook, 1991; Rogers, Dearing & Chang, 1991). In addition, when the media did cover the issue, it defined the problem less in terms of the lack of a cure for those already afflicted than as the absence of a vaccine that would control the spread of HIV to the general population. Media coverage was more inclined to reassure than criticize. Thus, until 1987 and the absence of the White House as a policy triggering mechanism, the policy agenda was seemingly unaffected. Colby and Cook (1991) posit that the policy agenda responded less to empirical indicators of the disease (the number of AIDS cases) or to the professional agenda (the number of medical articles on AIDS) than to the media agenda, the reasoning being that the political leaders responded to the public visibility the media had given AIDS earlier as affecting all groups in society and not just the "high risk" groups. Thus, in this period the heterosexualization of AIDS began to take place and what was discovered was the notion that everyone is susceptible to this virus, not just those who engage in "deviant" lifestyles.

After 1987, media coverage of AIDS slowly began to decline once again, and became more routine than in the previous years. Coverage was still framed in terms of lifestyle and scientific issues; however, the epidemic became more normalized with fewer references to imagery such as "gay plague" or it being the isolated disease of "others." For example, media coverage of the 1990 World AIDS Day focused specifically on women and children, two groups that had previously been the forgotten victims of AIDS. Now, one would see stories in the newspapers of the dangers AIDS posed to the reproductive lifestyle.

The findings of the literature on American media coverage of AIDS seem to apply to Anthony Downs' theory of "issue attention cycle" (Downs, 1972).

Downs suggests that the rise, peak, and decline of interest in a policy issue is subject to its importance or its "crisis status." Once the media has bored the public with the issue, its attention will slowly decline. According to the literature, such is the case of AIDS in American media coverage in the 1980s.

To summarize the literature on the American media coverage of AIDS, there is a cyclical dimension to AIDS reporting from 1981 to 1987 that eventually gives way to a more routine, event-driven coverage in the late 1980s and early 1990s.

AIDS COVERAGE IN SIX AMERICAN NEWSPAPERS 1981 TO 1994

Methodology

Much of the analysis that has been undertaken on the American media does not go beyond 1989 in its empirical data analysis and from this, one must surmise much of what is going on in the early years of the 1990s. Also, in large part, most of the analyses are of mixed media studies or network television coverage. The sole focus of this particular study is daily newspaper coverage. Newspaper coverage from 1981 to 1989 was examined to see if the findings of the existing literature apply. The years between 1990 to 1994 were then examined to discern and evaluate any new patterns or trends. Much of the methodology for this study has been suggested by previous research such as Rogers, Dearing, and Chang (1991). In large part, this is due to the need to verify that other research findings are reflected in the newspaper coverage for the same time period.

In this analysis, the mass media is represented by six major daily newspapers: *The New York Times*, the *Wall Street Journal*, the *Washington Post*, the *Chicago Tribune*, the *Los Angeles Times*, and the *San Francisco Chronicle*. These six were chosen for the following reasons. Firstly, these six combined most closely approximate a national newspaper media in the United States. Secondly, they are published in cities in which there has always been a heavy concentration of AIDS cases. Thirdly, the *Washington Post* was included also because of its crucial role in reporting national political events, including federal government policy. Fourthly, the *Wall Street Journal* was included because of its prominence in the business community and the perception of its general conservative viewpoints.[3] A longitudinal content analysis of the six newspapers was undertaken for the period beginning in January 1981 and ending in July 1994.

News Coverage Across the Six Newspapers

From January 1981 to July 1994, the six newspapers carried a total of 17,082 stories about AIDS. To see whether AIDS stories are disappearing from the media, despite the continuing growth in numbers of people infected, we

TABLE 5–1   Consistency of News Coverage Across Six Newspapers

Newspaper	No. of Stories 1981–1987	% of Total	No. of Stories 1988–1994	% of Total	Total 1981–1994	(%)
The New York Times	1817	24.7	3058	31.4	4875	28.5
San Francisco Chronicle	2013	27.4	1825	18.8	3838	22.5
Washington Post	1130	15.4	1507	15.5	2637	15.4
Los Angeles Times	1039	14.1	1519	15.6	2558	15.0
Chicago Tribune	998	13.5	1017	10.5	2015	11.8
Wall Street Journal	353	4.8	806	8.3	1159	6.8

divided the period 1981 to 1994 into two. Analysis shows that if one contrasts 1981–1987 (when the literature says coverage peaked) with 1988–1994, more stories actually appeared in the latter period. From 1981 to 1987, 7,350 stories were published in the six newspapers; this compares with 9,732 in the 1988–1994 period. Table 5–1 represents a breakdown by newspaper of the coverage. From the table we can see that with the exception of the *San Francisco Chronicle*, all papers increased their coverage in the 1988–1994 period compared with 1981–1987. Interestingly, when one considers how effected the city of San Francisco has been in the number of infected cases and AIDS deaths, the *San Francisco Chronicle's* coverage actually decreased. *The New York Times* and *Wall Street Journal* significantly increased the number of stories they covered in the latter period, whereas the three remaining papers witnessed more gradual increases. Table 5–1 also shows that out of all the newspapers, the *Wall Street Journal* had significantly less coverage and *The New York Times* more coverage for the entire 1981–1994 period.

The decrease in coverage in the San Francisco paper seems to suggest Downs' issue attention cycle holding true. Of all the cities, San Francisco, with its large homosexual population, has suffered heavily from the onset of the epidemic. Thus, we could argue that, to the general public of San Francisco, the AIDS issue is no longer news, but just a medical problem with which the city has to live. It is this that is reflected by the *San Francisco Chronicle's* coverage.

When we look at the number of stories by year we see a trend emerging (Figure 1). The highest number of stories in any given year appeared in 1987, which supports the findings in other media studies. However, since 1990 there has been a gradual decline in the number of stories appearing in the six papers. In 1987 there was a total of 3,324 stories; this compares to 877 in 1993 and 453 stories for the first seven months of 1994.

Figure 1 supports the sentiments expressed at the 1994 Unity Forum that old news may be no news and that AIDS stories are, indeed, fast disappearing from the newspapers despite the fact that each year in the 1990s we have experienced a growth in the number of newly diagnosed AIDS cases. We confirmed this by correlating the number of reported AIDS cases with the number of stories published while controlling for year. The analysis shows a –.51 correlation; this means that as the number of cases increased yearly, the number of published stories per year declined. According to federal health agency figures released in November 1994, the annual growth of the AIDS epidemic in the United States for 1992–1993 was three percent. Admittedly, this is the slowest growth since 1981, but the number of cases is still incredibly high (Table 5–2). It appears that not only is Downs' theory applicable, but that as the growth rate slows, so does the amount of media coverage.

The number of news stories about AIDS across time in each of the six newspapers are highly correlated. When one newspaper carried a high number of stories about AIDS, so did the others. The highest correlation was .94 between the coverage in *The New York Times* and the *Los Angeles Times*, and the lowest correlation was .73 between the number of stories that appeared in the *San Francisco Chronicle* and the *Washington Post.* The second lowest correlation, .84, was between *The New York Times* and the *San Francisco Chronicle*, in spite of the fact that both papers carry the most number of stories over time. We can conclude, therefore, that AIDS was treated with a certain degree of concurrence in the 1981 to 1994 time period.

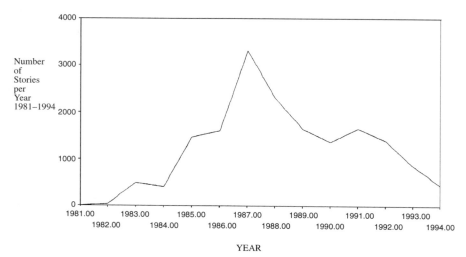

FIGURE 1. Number of AIDS stories per year, 1981–1994.

TABLE 5–2 Number of Reported AIDS
Cases in the United States 1981–93

Year	No. of Cases
1981	189
1982	650
1983	2,103
1984	4,515
1985	8,323
1986	13,280
1987	21,334
1988	32,060
1989	35,197
1990	43,319
1991	44,923
1992	49,016
1993	105,990

Source: CDC Annual Reports 1982–1984.

The Role of *The New York Times*

Numerous studies have been conducted that have shown the prominence and influence of *The New York Times*, as both a news source and agenda setter for various scientific issues (Ploughman, 1984; Mazur, 1987). To see whether this was also true on the AIDS issue, we compared *The New York Times* to the other five papers in terms of their AIDS coverage. Analysis shows that *The New York Times* outpaced the other newspapers in nine of the years under examination (1981, 1987, 1988, 1989, 1990, 1991, 1992, 1993, 1994) in terms of the total number of stories per annum. When *The New York Times* coverage is compared on a monthly basis with the five other newspapers, a clear pattern emerges. Despite being the paper that "broke" the AIDS story in January 1981, *The New York Times* was outpaced for the first forty-eight months of the period under examination. From January 1981 to December 1984 *The New York Times* only carried more stories than the other five papers in three months (January 1981, June and July 1983). In one other month (November 1983), it tied with the *San Francisco Chronicle* for the highest number of stories published. Thus, in the first four years of the epidemic, *The New York Times* was obviously neither an influential news source nor agenda setter on the AIDS issue. That role fell to the *San Francisco Chronicle*.

From January 1985 to December 1989 *The New York Times* published more news stories then its five competitors in twenty-eight months. In the peak year of coverage, 1987, the *Times* published the highest number of stories on the issue for nine months of the year. We can conclude that in the period from 1985 to 1989, *The New York Times* does start to emerge as an agenda setter and influential news source. It is from January 1990 to July 1994 that *The New York Times* emerges as the single most important news source and dominant agenda setter on the issue of AIDS. In only one month of the 1990s (June 1990), did the *Times* carry fewer stories about AIDS than the other five papers. Thus, the pattern we can discern is one in which *The New York Times* did not take an aggressive, agenda-setting role until the AIDS issue was perceived to be a crisis for society as a whole rather than for marginalized groups. In other words, when AIDS was no longer perceived to be a "gay plague," the *Times* became an incredibly aggressive, agenda-setting actor. This conclusion is consistent with the findings of studies of *The New York Times'* coverage on issues such as toxic waste and radon (Ploughman, 1984; Mazur, 1987). Such lethargy on the part of the *Times* is attributed in such studies to a lack of general public interest on the issue.

Cycles of Coverage

As stated earlier, the literature on the American media coverage of the AIDS issue suggests peaks of coverage. Most authors agree with Rogers, Dearing, and Chang (1991) that there are three peaks. The first peak occurs in May 1983 with the Fauci article, the second peak occurs in 1985 and is associated with Rock Hudson and Ryan White, and the third peak occurs in 1987 with the Reagan acknowledgment of the epidemic and federal government announcements on testing and screening policies. Analysis of the data shows that the three peaks are also common to the six newspapers in our study; however, as shown in Figure 1, a fourth peak occurs in 1991. This can be associated with the announcement by Earvin "Magic" Johnson of his HIV-positive status in that year. This fourth peak further exemplifies Downs' notion of the issue attention cycle. Thus, in 1991 with Johnson's announcement, not only is there an increase in the number of stories about the epidemic from the previous year, but the total number of stories for 1991 (1667) is the third highest for the entire thirteen years under examination (Figure 2). The Johnson announcement also further establishes the heterosexualization of the disease (Pollock, 1993). Figure 2 shows that once Johnson's plight faded in controversy, so did media coverage.

Types of AIDS Stories Published

This study uses a categorization scheme used by Rogers, Dearing, and Chang (1991, p. 19). These authors used a thirteen category scheme that divided stories into subissues. We have added an additional two categories and thus, all AIDS stories were placed into one of fifteen possible categories (1 through 13 are Rogers et al.'s; 14 and 15 are the additional categories). The categories are as follows:

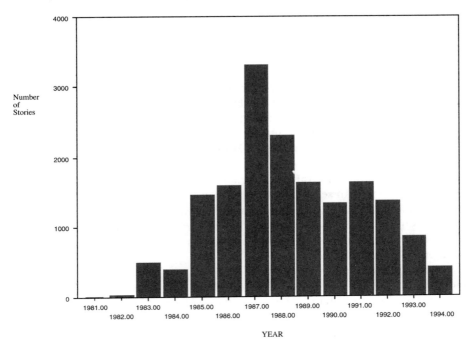

YEAR

FIGURE 2. Number of AIDS stories by year, 1981–1994.

Category name	Definition
1. Children with AIDS	News stories about children with AIDS.
2. Public figures	News stories about publicly recognized individuals with AIDS.
3. Epidemic	News stories reporting statistical facts about AIDS.
4. Biomedical	News stories about scientific findings on AIDS.
5. Prevention	News stories about methods to stop the spread of AIDS.
6. Discrimination	News stories reporting unfair treatment of people with AIDS.
7. People's help	News stories about community-based responses, i.e., nongovernmental activities.
8. Government policy	News stories about governmental action.
9. Civil rights	News stories about civil rights issues related to AIDS.
10. Ethics	News stories about immoral or irresponsible aspects of AIDS behavior.
11. Human interest	News stories describing people with AIDS as victims.
12. Poll results	News stories based on poll results about AIDS
13. Others	———

14. Heterosexualization   News stories about the increasing risks to
                            heterosexuals.
15. Gay plague   News stories associating AIDS with the gay
                            lifestyle.

Coding of the 17,082 stories was carried out by two coders with an overall intercoder agreement of 100 percent. Figure 3 shows the number of news stories for each of the fifteen categories for the 1981 to 1994 period. Two categories, biomedical and human interest, account for approximately 44 percent of all stories in the period (Figure 3). Human interest stories account overall for more stories than any other type of category.

Table 5–3 shows the ranking of each issue category from 1981 to 1994. From the table we can see that little attention has been paid to issues such as civil rights and ethics. Also, despite what the literature reports about the heavy emphasis of the media's coverage of AIDS as a gay plague, this does not hold true for the six newspapers in our analysis of number of stories that the papers have published in the period.

However, the analysis does show that this type of story was more common in 1981 to 1987 than in the 1988 to 1994 period, which is what one would expect. We also see a sharp increase in the number of stories of nongovernmental responses from the first period to the second period. This is perhaps

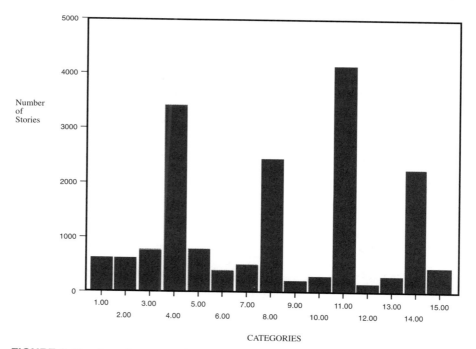

FIGURE 3. Number of news stories per issue category, 1981–1994.

TABLE 5–3 Issue Category Ranking by Number of Stories, 1981–94

Category	No. of Stories 1981–1987		No. of Stories 1988–1994		No. of Stories 1981–1994	
Human interest	1641	(22.3%)	2481	(25.5%)	4122	(24.1%)
Biomedical	1474	(20.0%)	1929	(19.8%)	3403	(19.9%)
Govt. policy	1076	(14.6%)	1347	(13.8%)	2423	(14.2%)
Others	710	(9.7%)	1537	(15.8%)	2249	(13.2%)
Prevention	423	(5.8%)	342	(3.5%)	765	(4.5%)
Epidemic	439	(6.0%)	314	(3.2%)	753	(4.4%)
Children	349	(4.7%)	249	(2.6%)	598	(3.5%)
Public figures	218	(3.0%)	365	(3.8%)	583	(3.4%)
People's help	113	(1.5%)	379	(3.9%)	462	(2.9%)
Gay plague	181	(2.5%)	236	(2.4%)	417	(2.4%)
Discrimination	222	(3.0%)	168	(1.7%)	390	(2.3%)
Heterosexualiz.	186	(2.5%)	94	(1.0%)	280	(1.6%)
Ethics	150	(2.0%)	127	(1.3%)	277	(1.6%)
Civil rights	99	(1.3%)	98	(1.0%)	197	(1.2%)
Poll results	69	(0.9%)	66	(0.7%)	133	(0.8%)
Total	7,350	(100.0%)	9,732	(100.0%)	17,082	(100.0%)

caused by the absence of a national AIDS policy in the United States and the need for an activist community response (Theodoulou, 1996).

Analysis shows substantial correlations among the number of stories per year for each of the fifteen categories for each of the six newspapers. The range being .26 to .97, with an average of approximately .63, or 39 percent of the variance explained. The general pattern that emerges from the data for the 1981 to 1994 period is that coverage of the fifteen subissue categories are consistent over time (Figure 4). Analysis demonstrates that an issue rises, falls, and then rises again, as other subissues gain and then lose media coverage.

As there are four peaks in overall media coverage, Figure 4 shows that there are also peaks in the number of stories about each issue category. Thus, each category has more stories in 1983, 1985, 1987, and 1991 than in other years.

Relationship of News Coverage to the Policy Agenda

We are using the number of stories published in the six newspapers in the time period under study as a measure of the media agenda. The policy agenda is measured as the annual amount of federal funds for AIDS research, education, and testing. Once again, this is a measure that has been used by other authors (Rogers, Dearing & Chang, 1991, p. 24). Although federal funds were spent as early as 1982, through funding reallocations within the CDC, the U.S. Congress first officially allocated federal

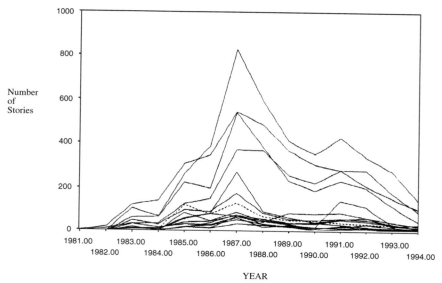

FIGURE 4. Coverage by issue category, 1981–1994.

funds under the label "AIDS research, education, and testing" in 1983. Until 1990, the U.S. Congress has approximately doubled AIDS funding each year; however, since 1991, there has been a decline in federal funding reaching $1.48 billion in 1994, which is approximately $.12 billion less then 1990 funding.

The media agenda on AIDS and the policy agenda show a statistically significant correlation of .32 (P < .5). Thus, as the number of stories increases, so does federal funding on AIDS. The media agenda does affect the policy agenda over time, although the AIDS media agenda explains only 10 percent of the variance in the policy agenda.

Number of AIDS Cases

If we take the number of reported AIDS cases (this figure does not include reported HIV-positive infections) as a real world indicator of the epidemic, we see that there has been a continual growth in the total number of reported AIDS cases in the United States (Figure 5). Data show that the annual number of reported AIDS cases in the United States is increasing. However, the relationship of the number of AIDS cases to the media agenda and the policy agenda can be seen to be weak. The number of AIDS cases explains approximately 4.8 percent of the variance in the media agenda over time, while the number of AIDS cases explains about 10 percent of the variance in the policy agenda. Although both are statistically significant, their level of significance is not particularly high.

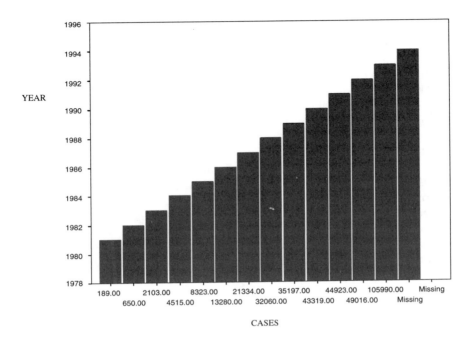

FIGURE 5. Annual number of AIDS cases 1981–1994.

SUMMARY AND INTERPRETATION

This paper has examined the level of coverage in six national newspapers in America and the relationship of the media agenda to the policy agenda on the issue of AIDS. The newspapers were found to be highly correlated in their coverage of AIDS during the 1981 to 1994 time period. Despite the growth in the number of AIDS cases, the issue has never ranked high on the media agenda. For example, it was not ranked a top ten news story until 1985 by the Associated Press. This slow media response was due in part to the failure of *The New York Times* to act as a significant news source and agenda setter on the issue, and also in part to President Reagan's late acknowledgment of the epidemic (Perrow & Guillen, 1990, p. 51; Theodoulou, 1996). Thus the White House failed to move the AIDS issue onto the media agenda.

In terms of coverage, there are four distinct peaks of coverage: 1983, 1985, 1987, and 1991. More stories appeared in the 1988 to 1994 period than in 1981 to 1987, although each year in the 1990s we have witnessed a decline in coverage. *The New York Times* after a slow start has, since 1990, become the dominant news source and agenda setter on the issue of AIDS. When we look at the thirteen years of the AIDS epidemic, we see that Anthony Downs' issue attention cycle is supported by the data.

The data also show that there is a relationship between the media agenda and the policy agenda, although not to the degree that some might believe. Finally, in terms of the impact of the number of AIDS cases, there is a weak relationship between the numbers infected and the media and policy agendas (Figure 6).

The data do not strongly support the argument that the media has perpetuated a continuing ideology of AIDS homophobia in terms of the number of stories reported. However, one of the shortcomings of this study is that we have looked at total numbers rather than actual content of story. Many would argue that the media's account of the epidemic is in fact one of discriminatory statements and subtle homophobic marginalization of the plight of homosexuals with AIDS compared with other people living with the disease. Finally, it does appear that the media has helped to construct AIDS as a scientific issue.

Our analysis suggests that the urgency surrounding the AIDS epidemic has ebbed. In the 1990s AIDS is viewed as just another intractable problem, like homelessness or drug abuse (Kirp & Bayer, 1992, p. 381). From the data we can observe that AIDS has become a stable matter for the media. This fact has far-reaching implications for the manner in which societal attitudes towards the issue have changed over time. It implies that AIDS is losing its intensity and prominence as a major health issue, along with its newsworthiness, despite the growing numbers of infected.

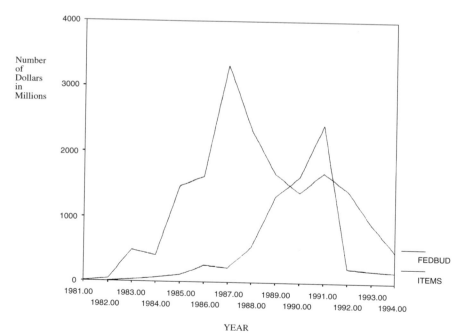

FIGURE 6. Media agenda relationship to policy agenda.

It is likely that news coverage will continue to diminish in both intensity and quantity, unless a new dimension or controversy is added to the disease. The consequences of the failure of the media to see AIDS as a newsworthy issue are many. Firstly, it will lead to a decline in the interest and support of the general public. Secondly, it will be difficult to maintain high levels of awareness, thus thwarting education and prevention programs. Lastly, there will be less pressure on the American political leadership to improve its performance in the areas of funding, research, and overall policy.

The chronology and shape of the media response provides a clear example of Anthony Downs' issue attention cycle. The shape of media coverage also conforms to analyses of media coverage of other health issues (Ives, 1986, Berridge, 1991). Finally, in policy terms it appears that the media has reinforced the consensual reaction to AIDS (Street, 1988). AIDS attracted attention when it first appeared, but after the immediate controversy what emerged was typical incremental policymaking. Professional and political consensus was the key to policymaking; and AIDS, according to Fox, Day, and Klein (1989); Day and Klein (1990); and Street (1988), has been dealt with according to existing conceptual models. The "gay plague" era of press coverage was simply part of the original controversy period and must be understood as part of the overall ideological environment of that time.

NOTES

1. Throughout this study AIDS is used as shorthand for the more encompassing term human immunodeficiency virus (HIV)/AIDS, except where this usage would cause confusion or is strictly incorrect. For example, individuals are described as HIV antibody positive rather than AIDS positive when they have not developed any of the symptoms of AIDS but have antibodies for the HIV.

2. The forum is an annual conference of newspaper reporters and was held in Atlanta, Georgia in the summer of 1994.

3. Increasingly, as the epidemic has spread, its impact on the economies of the world has become clear.

REFERENCES

Abraham, C., Sheeran, P. Abrams, D., et al. (1991). Young people learning about AIDS: a study of beliefs and information sources. *Health Education Research*, 6.1: pp. 19–29.

Adams, J. (1989). *AIDS: The HIV Myth*. New York: St. Martin's Press.

Albert, E. (1986a). Acquired immune deficiency syndrome: the victim and the press. *Studies in Communication*, 3: pp. 135–58.

———. (1986b). Illness and deviance: the response of the press to AIDS, in Feldman, D.A., & Johnson, T.M., eds., *The Social Dimensions of AIDS: Methods and Theory.* New York: Praeger.

Austin, S.B. (1990). AIDS and Africa: U.S. media and racist fantasy. *Cultural Critique*, 14: pp. 129–41.

Baker, A. (1986). The portrayal of AIDS in the media: an analysis of articles in the New York Times, in Feldman, D.A., & Johnson, T.M., eds., *The Social Dimensions of AIDS: Methods and Theory.* New York: Praeger.

Beharrell, P. (March 1991). Information or myth?, unpublished paper presented to British Sociological Conference, Manchester.

———. (1993). AIDS and the British press, in Eldridge, J.E.T., ed., *Getting the Message.* London: Routledge.

Berridge, V. (1991). AIDS, the media and health policy. *Health Education Journal*, 50.4: pp. 179–85.

Boffin, T., & Gupta, S., eds. (1990). *Ecstatic Antibodies.* London: Rivers Oram Press.

Bray, F., & Chapman, S. (1991). Community knowledge, attitudes, and media recall about AIDS, Sydney 1988 & 1989. *Australian Journal of Public Health*, 15.2: pp. 107–13.

Carducci, A., Frasca, M., Matteelli, M., et al. (1990). AIDS information and Italian youth: a survey on military recruits. *AIDS Education and Prevention*, 15.23: pp. 181–90.

Clarke, J.N. (1991). Media portrayal of a disease from the medical, political economy, and lifestyle perspectives. *Quantitative Health Research*, 1.3: pp. 287–308.

———. (1992). Cancer, heart disease, and AIDS: what do the media tell us about these diseases? *Health Communications*, 4.2: pp. 105–20.

Colby, T., & Cook, D. (1991). Epidemics and agendas: the politics of nightly news coverage of AIDS. *Journal of Health, Politics, Policy and Law*, 16.2: pp. 215–49.

Crimp, D. (1992). Portraits of people with AIDS, in Grossberg, L., Nelson, C., & Treichler, P.A., eds., *Cultural Studies.* New York: Routledge.

Cunningham, I. (1989). The public controversies of AIDS in Puerto Rico. *Social Science and Medicine*, 29.4: pp. 545–53.

Day, P., & Klein, R. (1990). Interpreting the unexpected: the case of AIDS, policy making in Britain. *Journal of Public Policy*, 9: pp. 337–53.

Dolan, R., Corber, S., & Zacow, R. (1990). A survey of knowledge and attitudes with regard to AIDS among grade 7 and 8 students in Ottawa-Carlton. *Canadian Journal of Public Health*, 81: pp. 135–38.

Downs, A. (1972). Up and down with ecology—'the issue attention cycle'. *Public Interest*, 32: pp. 38–50.

Feldman, D., & Johnson, T.M., eds. (1986). *The Social Dimensions of AIDS: Methods and Theory.* New York: Praeger.

Fox, D., Day, P., & Klein, R. (1989). The power of professionalism: AIDS in Britain, Sweden, and the United States. *Daedalus*, 118: pp. 93–112.

French, R., & Duffin, R. (1986). Mossies could spread AIDS. *Australian Media References on AIDS, 1981–1985.* Sydney, Gay History Project.

Herzlich, C., & Pierret, J. (1989). The construction of a social phenomenon: AIDS in the French press. *Social Science and Medicine*, 29.11: pp. 1235–42.

Hughey, J., Norton, R., and Sullivan-Norton, C. (1989). Insidious metaphors and the changing meaning of AIDS. *AIDS and Public Policy Journal*, 4.1: pp. 56–67.

Ives, R. (1986). The rise and fall of the solvents panic. *Druglink*, 1.4: pp. 10–12.

Jones, J.W. (1992). Discourses on and of AIDS in West Germany, 1986–1990. *Journal of the History of Sexuality*, 2.3: pp. 439–68.

King, D. (1990). 'Prostitutes as pariah in the age of AIDS': a content analysis of coverage of women prostitutes in the New York Times and the Washington Post September 1985–April 1988. *Women and Health*, 16.3–4: pp. 155–76.

Kirp, D.L., & Bayer, R. (1992). The second decade of AIDS: the end of exceptional-ism?, in Kirp, D.L., & Bayer, R., eds., *AIDS in the Industrialized Democracies: Passions, Politics, and Policies*. New Brunswick: Rutgers University Press.

Kitzinger, J. (1990). Audience understandings of AIDS media messages: a discussion of methods. *Sociology of Health and Illness*, 12.3: pp. 320–35.

Kitzinger, J., & Miller, D. (1991). *In Black and White: A Preliminary Report on the Role of the Media in Audience Understandings of 'African AIDS'*. Glasgow: AIDS Media Research Project.

Lupton, D. (1994). *Moral Threats and Dangerous Desires: AIDS in the News Media*. Bristol, PA: Taylor & Francis.

Mangaliman, Jesse. (August 1994). Unity Forum Conference Proceedings.

Mazur, A. (1987). Putting radon on the public risk agenda. *Science, Technology and Human Values*, 12.3–4: pp. 86–93.

Murray, J. (1991). Bad press: representations of AIDS in the media. *Cultural Studies from Birmingham*, 1: pp. 29–51.

Nelkin, D. (1991). AIDS and the news media. *Milbank Quarterly*, 69.2: pp. 293–306.

Penny, R. (1988). Changing perspectives 1982–1988. *Report of the Third National Conference on AIDS, Living with AIDS, Toward the Year 2000*, Hobart, 4–6, Department of Community Services and Health, pp. 76–8. Canberra: Australian Government Printing Service.

Perrow, C., & Guillen, M. (1990). *The AIDS Disaster: The Failure of Organizations in New York and the Nation*. New Haven, Conn.: Yale University Press.

Ploughman, P. (1984). The creation of newsworthy events: an analysis of newspaper coverage of the man made disaster at Love Canal. (Ph.D. diss., State University of New York at Buffalo.)

Pollock, P., Lillie, S., & Vittes, M. (March 1993). On the nature and dynamics of social construction: the case of AIDS. *Social Science Quarterly*, pp. 123–35.

Rogers, M., Dearing, J.W., & Chang S. (1991). AIDS in the 1990's: the agenda setting process for a public issue. *Journalism Monographs*, No. 126, Association for Education in Journalism and Mass Communication.

Ross, M.W., & Carson, J.A. (1988). Effectiveness of distribution of information on AIDS: a national study of six media in Australia. *New York State Journal of Medicine*, pp. 239–41.

Ross, M.W. (1989). Psychosocial ethical aspects of AIDS. *Journal of Medical Ethics*, 15: pp. 74–81.

Street, J. (1988). British government policy on AIDS. *Parliamentary Affairs*, 41: pp. 490–508.

Theodoulou, S.Z. (1996). This volume, part 1, chapter 1.

Tulloch, J. (1989). Australian television and the representation of AIDS. *Australian Journal of Communication*, 16: pp. 101–24.

——. (1992). Using TV in HIV/AIDS education: production and audience cultures. *Media Information Australia*, 65: pp. 28–35.

Wellings, K. (1988). Perceptions of risk-media treatment of AIDS, in Aggleton, P., & Homan, H., eds. *Social Aspects of AIDS*. Basingstroke: U.K. Falmer Press.

White, Phillips, Pitt, et al. (1988). Adolescents' perceptions of AIDS. *Health Education Journal*, 47.4: pp. 117–27.

6

The Politics of Deservedness: The Ryan White Act and the Social Constructions of People with AIDS

Mark C. Donovan

Since the appearance of acquired immune deficiency syndrome (AIDS) in the United States, the epidemic has been characterized variously as a "plague," a "holocaust," and a "natural disaster." Though skeptics may be inclined to dismiss such characterizations as hyperbole, the statistics are sobering. As of June 1994, the Centers for Disease Control and Prevention (CDC) reported that 400,000 Americans had been diagnosed with AIDS and more than 240,000 had died—more than three times the number of American deaths in the Vietnam war (CDC, 1994). AIDS has become the third leading cause of death among adults between the ages of 25 to 44 nationwide and it is estimated that one in 250 persons in the United States is infected with human immunodeficiency virus, (HIV), the virus thought to cause AIDS (CDC, 1993). Clearly the many challenges posed by the HIV/AIDS crisis are not going away anytime soon.

Students of United States politics and policy must understand the important role that perceptions of deservedness play in both the design of public policy and the public justifications lawmakers offer for their policy choices. The governmental response to the AIDS epidemic nicely illustrates the link between political language and public policy—a link that does much to explain inequalities in the distribution of benefits and burdens. In this chapter I approach AIDS policymaking from a perspective that emphasizes

Donovan, Mark C. "The Politics of Deservedness: The Ryan White Act and the Social Constructions of People with AIDS," *Policy Studies Review*, Vol. 12, No. 3/4 Autumn/Winter, 1993. Reprinted by permission.

how socially constructed stereotypes of different groups of people with AIDS are reflected in the shape of federal policy.

THE SOCIAL CONSTRUCTION PERSPECTIVE

The connection between pervasive stereotypes and public policymaking is at the center of a recent framework for social construction analysis proposed by Schneider and Ingram (1993). They present a parsimonious model of policy-making that holds that both the justifications for and the substance of public policies can be broadly predicted by understanding the social construction and political power of the groups being targeted by a given policy. In this section the Schneider and Ingram perspective is outlined and in the next the factors that have influenced the various social constructions of people with AIDS (PWAs) are discussed.

Schneider and Ingram's starting point is that within a society, identifiable groups of individuals—target populations—are imbued with culturally constructed positive or negative images. These images, in turn, influence the types of policy benefits and burdens lawmakers are willing to aim at those groups. When a concern for re-election drives the decisions of lawmakers, public officials must be certain that their policy choices—including the selection of target populations to receive benefits and burdens—will maximize their electoral advantage. Therefore, public officials can be expected to make policies that treat groups in ways that conform to dominant societal stereotypes. For the most part this means that politicians attempt to bestow benefits on positively constructed groups and burdens on negatively constructed groups.

But there is a catch. In addition to the social image of a particular group, politicians must also be aware of the relative political power of various populations. Powerful positively constructed populations and powerless negatively constructed populations represent congruent political ideal types. Politicians can bolster their popularity and electoral advantage by conferring benefits on advantaged groups and dumping burdens on deviant ones. When the powerless are positively constructed or, more troublesome for the politician, when powerful groups are negatively constructed, policy decisions become less straightforward. Although policymakers must present a "believable causal logic connecting the various aspects of the policy design to desired outcomes" there are often multiple logics available (Schneider and Ingram, 1993: 336). Legislators can thus be expected to exploit rhetorical strategies that maximize the benefits and minimize the burdens targeted at preferred groups.

Schneider and Ingram develop a typology of target populations that simplifies a complex reality by holding that four key types of target populations are defined by the intersections of social construction (dichotomized as positive or negative) and political power (dichotomized as high or low). This typology is reproduced in Table 6–1. "Advantaged" groups having a relatively large degree of political power and predominantly positive image to society are more likely to receive benefits when targeted by public policies. As a result of both direct political power and the symbolic leverage accompanying their popular image, these groups have a relatively high degree of control over the shape of policies selecting them as targets. "Contending" groups having a relatively large degree of political power but a predominantly negative public image have little control over the distribution of policy benefits, but some degree of control over the shape of policy burdens. In view of their negative public construction they are likely to be the subject of at least some symbolic burdens while any benefits conferred by a policy will generally be delivered out of the public eye, or will be justified with an attempt to generalize the benefit, arguing, for example, that it is "in the national interest" to grant such a group a policy benefit.

This typology of target populations is completed by two additional categories of groups, each possessing little political power. "Dependent" groups are more likely to receive burdens rather than benefits, but given their prevailing positive construction these groups may be able to exert some leverage on the policy process in order to be targeted for policy benefits. These benefits, though, are likely to be symbolic rather than substantive. "Deviant" groups are also likely to receive burdens rather than benefits, but, lacking power and a positive construction, deviants are unlikely to be able to influence policy in ways beneficial to them. Under Schneider and Ingram's schema, people with AIDS fit into either the dependent or deviant cell. Women, children, hemophiliacs, and blood transfusion recipients are generally constructed as dependents, while gays and injection drug users (IDUs) are labeled deviant. It needs to be stressed that these are not hard and fast designations. The position of gays in the matrix of target populations has shifted over time as the gay community politically mobilized its members, increasing

TABLE 6–1 Typology Social Constructions with Hypothetical Target Populations

	Social Construction	
Power	Positive	Negative
Powerful	Advantaged	Contenders
	The Elderly	The rich
	Business	Big unions
Powerless	Dependents	Deviants
	Children	Criminals
	Disabled	Drug addicts

Adapted from Schneider and Ingram, 1993, Figure 1.

its political profile but not eradicating the negative constructions of gay men with AIDS.

Schneider and Ingram's typology is useful because it provides a framework for systematically unpacking key influences on the policymaking process. Furthermore, it helps to explain inequalities in the distribution of benefits and burdens to different groups and illustrates the important connections between political language and public policy. Such an analysis is especially useful in a case such as AIDS where rhetoric is so charged and the stakes so high. In the next section, I examine the factors that have shaped the social constructions of PWAs and attempt to convince the reader that throughout the AIDS epidemic people with AIDS have been publicly grouped and characterized in ways that have important implications for how they are regarded by the public. I then use the Schneider and Ingram framework to guide the analysis of a landmark piece of AIDS legislation, the Ryan White Act, in which the potent symbolism of "dependent" populations and the difficult position of "deviant" populations is clear.

THE SOCIAL CONSTRUCTION OF PEOPLE WITH AIDS

To note that AIDS is a socially constructed phenomenon is not to deny the reality that HIV is a infectious virus that most often results in the death of those it infects. Rather, the point is to focus more clearly on the ways in which historical, technical, and cultural forces have injected our representation of this condition with certain qualities and to investigate the effect of this representation on policy design. While the social construction of images of AIDS and PWAs is a complex and dynamic process, three sources of these constructions stand out. First, the discovery of AIDS set in motion historically familiar responses to the epidemic. Second, the definition and categorization of HIV/AIDS by medical professionals determined in important ways how target populations would be identified. Third, latent cultural stereotypes of the groups to which many PWAs can be said to belong have had a profound influence on the shape of policies targeted at these groups. After discussing each of these three sources in greater detail, I examine how the initial constructions of PWAs changed over time and influenced the debate over AIDS policy.

A major source of the construction of AIDS and PWAs has been the familiar historical script of an epidemic. Thus conceived, the initial public response to the AIDS epidemic was on one level a decidedly traditional one. The response followed an archetypal pattern beginning with the slow revelation of the existence of the epidemic, progressing to a stage at which infection was equated with moral failing, and ultimately eliciting a policy response intended to restore the pre-epidemic order (Rosenberg, 1989; see also Hughes, 1993). This patterned response was undoubtedly accelerated by modern communications technology. One pair of observers dubbed this mass-mediated epidemic the first "living-room epidemic" where the revelation of a spreading contagion came not with a firsthand exposure to the epidemic's effects but through television images of AIDS sufferers (Cook & Colby, 1992). While public awareness of the epidemic occurred relatively early, the medium delivering the message probably served to reinforce the historically familiar public reaction of distancing oneself from the possibility of infection.

Secondly, the decisions and responses of professionals involved in AIDS policymaking also played a significant role in the construction of target populations. First, the determination of the official definition of AIDS by public health officials prompted a particular set of public responses to the epidemic. AIDS is not a disease, but rather a syndrome: an umbrella designation for a condition marked by an immune system destroyed by HIV and invaded by any of a number of opportunistic infections. To "have AIDS" means that a person has tested HIV+ and suffers from an infection on the list of "official" AIDS infections. The definition of AIDS underwent significant revisions in 1985, 1987, and 1993. The definition has substantive importance because it determines who qualifies for government benefits and serves to shape who, quite literally, becomes an AIDS statistic. These statistics, in turn, shape how elites and the public conceive of people with AIDS, and serve to both include and exclude different groups from policymakers' consideration. The most notable example is the failure of official AIDS definitions to include the gynecological manifestations of the syndrome thus excluding many women from the definition, limiting their access to services, and misstating the character of the epidemic (Corea, 1992). The *de facto* exclusion of women from the definition of AIDS further bolstered the early stereotypes of PWAs as gay men and IDUs, reinforcing skewed perceptions of the epidemic.

Even if the AIDS definition had been more inclusive from the beginning, the classification of AIDS as a sexually transmitted disease contributed in important ways to the dominant constructions of PWAs. Though HIV can be contracted in a variety of nonsexual ways, AIDS has been classified as a sexually transmitted disease rather than as a viral disease. Instead of labeling AIDS a viral disease such as Hepatitis B, which is transmittable in most of the same ways as HIV, AIDS has been categorized as a sexually transmitted disease (STD) much like syphilis or gonorrhea (Gilman, 1988: 247). This is significant because, as Allan Brandt notes in his social history of venereal disease in America, "Medical and social values continue to define venereal disease as a uniquely sinful disease, indeed, to transform the disease into an indication of moral decay" (Brandt, 1985: 186). Thus, the medical definition of AIDS as an STD practically insured that issues such as prevention and treatment would involve a policy debate centering on moral as well as medical judgments.

Clearly, the medical response to AIDS cannot be easily divorced from historically familiar responses that centered on placing blame. As Dorothy Nelkin and Sander Gilman note, the relationship between devastating disease and the compulsion to assign blame for the devastation is age-old. They write that, "Clinical categories . . . are frequently associated with specific groups— sometimes identified by race, sometimes by nationality or social class. In each case, blame for disease turns into a crusade against those who are feared or who, by being different, are viewed as a threat to the established social order" (Nelkin & Gilman 1991: 45). As with those infected during past epidemics, PWAs came to be seen as belonging to one of two groups. Most were regarded as blameworthy "carriers of AIDS," a much smaller number came to be viewed as the "innocent victims of AIDS."

The possible ramifications of such labeling can be seen historically in the federal response to syphilis at the beginning of this century. Syphilitic male soldiers were framed as the patriotic victims of disease-carrying prostitutes who, through their ostensibly willful infection of the fighting force, were implicitly collaborating with the enemy (Fee, 1988). Placing infected individuals into such moral categories has a clear influence on the policies aimed not just at infected individuals, but also at the groups to which these infected persons are said to belong. Prostitutes during World War I became seen as more than mere collaborators with the enemy, they were effectively identified as the enemy. Labeled "venereal carriers," more than 30,000 prostitutes were detained by Congressional order in government-sponsored institutions during World War I (Brandt, 1988). This policy response was echoed by elected officials confronting the AIDS epidemic when suggestions of the quarantining and mass firings of gays were reportedly discussed within the Reagan administration (Altman, 1986: 64).

Finally, while the historical scripts for responding to epidemics and the classification of AIDS as a sexually transmitted disease provided an almost unconsciously accepted set of social constructions of PWAs, the force of cultural stereotypes of the groups associated with HIV/AIDS—most notably the popular images of gay men and injection drug users—had a profound influence on the formation of policies to combat the epidemic. Public health officials initially dubbed what would come to be known as AIDS a "gay cancer" and then later "Gay related immune disorder (GRID)," choices that forged an early and lasting link between homosexuality and infection. As the public health establishment has distanced itself from emphasizing "risk group" and focused instead on "risk behaviors" PWAs have been categorized according to the probable context of HIV transmission—"homosexual sex," "illegal drug use," "blood transfusion," and so forth. While these designations may make sense for the purpose of collecting epidemiological data and targeting prevention efforts, they also serve to provide important cues to elites and the public about how to regard particular groups of PWAs. A 1983 *New York Times Magazine* article noted that, "The groups most recently found to be at risk for AIDS present a particularly poignant problem"; hemophiliacs, transfusion recipients, and babies were "innocent bystanders caught in the path of a new disease" (Brandt, 1988: 165). But the flipside of "innocence" is of course "guilt" and the construction of gays and IDUs as "guilty" was widely adopted in public rhetoric throughout the 1980s.

As noted above, the innocent/guilty dichotomy is a construction of the infected that predates the appearance of AIDS. The appearance of HIV/AIDS in already marginalized groups, though, reinforced this tendency to identify sickness with moral failing. One pair of observers notes that public stigmatization of homosexuality and drug use led many to adopt "the stand that *it is better to let the guilty die of AIDS than to risk encouraging extramarital sex or drug abuse among the still innocent* " (Perrow and Guillén, 1990: 8, emphasis in original).

This concern for the judgment of people with AIDS remained even in the face of contradictory evidence. Early studies confirming the heterosexual transmission of HIV came under attack from researchers who insisted that such results were the artifact of unreported homosexuality. It seemed so difficult to separate discussions of sexual practice from sexual identity that, unwilling to make such a distinction, one critic even went so far as to suggest that a man's visit to a female prostitute (presumably resulting in HIV transmission) should be thought of as a "quasihomosexual" act (Treichler, 1988: 205–208). The obsession with the sexual character of AIDS also served to drown out important trends in the epidemic. Daniel Fox observes that:

> In the early 1980s, when most media attention and most advocacy for policy focused on AIDS as a disease of homosexuals, hemophiliacs, and recipients of transfused blood, overwhelming statistical evidence revealed that the epidemic was a serious problem for blacks and Hispanics and that most of the people at risk of infection in these groups were of relatively low socioeconomic status. In 1982 . . . blacks and Hispanics comprised just under half of the males, almost 80 percent of the females, and almost two-thirds of the children diagnosed with the disease in the United States. (1992: 129)

Even as the public understanding of the epidemic has changed, it often still focuses on assessing the relative deservedness of PWAs. As one HIV+ woman notes, "If I tell you I was diagnosed with a terminal illness, the normal reaction is 'Oh, do you need anything? How are you feeling? If I say I have AIDS, the first question is 'How did you get it? What have you been doing?' " (Meredith, 1992: 231).

The contingent nature of the construction of PWA target populations is highlighted by crossnational comparisons. In the Netherlands, injection drug use is viewed not as deviant stigmatized behavior, but as a medical problem requiring intervention and treatment—"harm reduction" (Kirp & Bayer, 1992). In many northern European countries, constructions of PWAs have been "medicalized" rather than "moralized" (Perrow & Guillén, 1992: 7). In Japan, the first domestic AIDS cases to receive widespread media attention were placed in the context of heterosexual transmission leading to a different construction of PWAs than in the United States (Dearing, 1992). Since worldwide approximately 90 percent of new HIV infections result from heterosexual transmission and approximately 70 percent of all those infected are female (Hombs, 1992) the characterization of the epidemic in the United States as a plague of gays and drug users must be seen as more than just a particular reading of U.S. AIDS demographics. The U.S. reaction to AIDS also can be considered as a social problem whose construction draws heavily on historical patterns, technical decisions, and cultural images.

THE RYAN WHITE CARE ACT

The importance of taking into account the social constructions of target populations when examining public policy is bluntly illustrated by examining the Ryan White Comprehensive AIDS Resource Emergency (CARE) Act. Passed in 1990, the act was the first piece of comprehensive AIDS legislation designed to deliver treatment and care to PWAs. The way the act distributed burdens and benefits to various groups of PWAs supports Schneider and Ingram's typology of target populations and illuminates ways in which political constraints hamper the adoption of effective policies. Passage of the law was made possible by events that helped to broaden the public conception of who is at risk for HIV infection, which allowed lawmakers to argue that the act would take care of the "innocent victims" of AIDS—a rationale on which they overwhelmingly relied on in their public statements.

The conventional wisdom, expressed by journalist Randy Shilts (1987: 585) is "that there were two clear phases to the disease in the United States: there was AIDS before Rock Hudson and AIDS after." This common observation has been confirmed by Rogers, Dearing, and Chang (1991) who note that Hudson's 1985 disclosure that he was suffering from AIDS—rather than a change in the character of the epidemic or the introduction of new, substantive information about AIDS—led to a permanent increase in media attention to the disease. Kinsella (1989) similarly argues that media coverage of AIDS has been tied to the extent to which the threat to "mainstream" Americans was perceived to be increasing, rather than to empirical indicators such as the epidemic's death toll.

Though the Hudson announcement is commonly viewed as a milestone, emphasis also should be placed on the coverage of Ryan White's exclusion from school in Kokomo, Indiana and his successful battle to return to the classroom. The two media events occurred nearly simultaneously: the official Hudson announcement came on July 30, 1985, following weeks of speculation; the first Ryan White story appeared on network television the next day followed by several reports from all three networks in the month leading up to his return to school in August 1985 (Cook & Colby, 1992: 121). The increased media attention to AIDS that immediately followed this joint event consisted of more than just stories about the two figures—in fact, news stories about

Rock Hudson and Ryan White accounted together for less than half of the increase in news stories about AIDS. The event put AIDS on the media agenda and "changed the meaning of the issue of AIDS for media newspeople, and ultimately for the American people" (Rogers, Dearing & Chang, 1991: 13).

This change is significant because it led to a shift in the social construction of PWA target populations, and because it came about as a result of the media messages about Hudson and White that were incongruous with the dominant societal stereotype of a person with AIDS. The case of Hudson is particularly instructive because as a gay man one would not necessarily imagine that his announcement would force a reconsideration of PWAs. Paula Treichler has observed, though, that many in the media and public could not reconcile Hudson's masculine screen persona with news of his homosexuality. She suggests that news stories attempted to "normalize" Hudson and cites as an example a *USA Today* article on the event in which a man is quoted saying "I thought AIDS was a gay disease, but if Rock Hudson can get it, anyone can" (Treichler, 1988: 205, 249–50). For many, it seems, it was easier to think of AIDS as no longer just a "gay disease" than it was to reconcile deep stereotypes about homosexuality. For others, the sickness of such a prominent figure served to change thinking that labeled PWAs as "marginal."

The Ryan White story also served to reshuffle the prevailing construction of PWAs (see also Kirp, 1989). White, a hemophiliac, appeared on television as a relatively healthy looking young teen, and through his activism and many media appearances he became the personification of the message that "anyone can get AIDS." Still, the incongruity of a child with AIDS did not instantly dispel fears of AIDS and the accompanying stereotypes of PWAs. In a typographical error that seems to belie this confusion, one newspaper ran a photo of White in 1986 noting that he was a "homophiliac" (Gilman, 1988: 268). The Hudson/White media event created dissonance within the public discourse that led to social learning about AIDS. This and other incongruities between nongay, noninjection drug using PWAs and prevailing stereotypes did not lead to a reassessment of the negative construction of gays and IDUs with AIDS, but instead led to the creation of new target populations—"women with AIDS" and "children with AIDS."

This shift in public consciousness provided an opportunity for policy-makers to construct an AIDS policy that could deliver benefits to "deserving" target populations. Before this shift, lawmakers did not perceive the extension of care and treatment to PWAs as a defensible policy in light of the prevailing image of AIDS sufferers and their own focus on reelection. At the time the Ryan White Act was considered, PWA target populations were arrayed along the continuums of political power and positive/negative construction in a manner illustrated in Figure 1. The percent of the total PWAs represented by each group in 1990 is noted in parentheses in the figure. There is, of course, some overlapping membership between some groups (for instance, gay men who inject drugs). This arrangement of target populations is based on a review of a wide range of published analysis and commentary on the epidemic (see also Bayer, 1989; Crimp, 1987; Epstein, 1991; Grmek, 1990; Hughey, Norton, & Sullivan-Norton, 1989; MacKinnon, 1992; Presidential Commission on the Human Immunodeficiency Virus Epidemic, 1988; Price, 1992; Quam & Ford, 1990; Ron & Rogers, 1989; Wachter, 1992).

While the absolute position of groups is to some extent arbitrary, the relative position of each population is not. It is worth stressing that Figure 1 does not map PWA target populations onto the four social construction ideal types reviewed above and illustrated in Table 6–1; the figure presents the populations only in relation to one another. Injection drug users anchor the lower righthand corner of the space with an extremely negative image and no political power. The political mobilization of the gay community and an increasingly favorable (though still predominantly negative) public image is noted by the up and leftward movement of the gay community. Women and racial and ethnic minorities are located on the social construction continuum some-

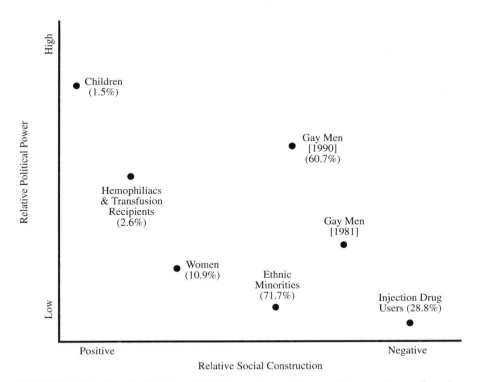

FIGURE 1. Relative distribution of PWA target populations with percentage of total AIDS cases by category, 1990. (*Source:* AIDS case data from National Research Council, 1993, pp. 44, 51, 55. Percentages sum to over 100% as a result of overlapping group membership.)

where between drug users and children as their infection still conveys to many evidence of a moral failing. They are positioned relatively low on the power continuum because as a group their political mobilization has lagged behind the gay community and advocates for children. Children, hemophiliacs, and blood transfusion recipients are all positively constructed. Children, by virtue of the political mobilization of pediatric AIDS lobbying groups and the prevailing sympathy for their plight, are the most politically powerful of these groups. In absolute terms, though, none of the PWA groups can be said to be politically powerful.

The House version of the Ryan White CARE Act (HR 4785) was sponsored by Henry Waxman (D-CA), the Senate version (S 2240) by Edward Kennedy (D-MA). Both bills passed with overwhelming bipartisan support, though the subsequent failure of the Congress to fully fund the act suggests that much of this support may have been purely symbolic. The House bill cleared the chamber on June 13, 1990 with a vote of 408–14. The Senate version passed a month earlier on May 16, 95–4. The markup period in the House Subcommittee on Health and the Environment, chaired by Waxman, and the floor debate in both houses was spent considering a variety of restrictive amendments offered by Republican lawmakers. Amendments requiring states to develop partner notification programs and forbidding the use of grants to fund needle exchange programs were adopted in response to more restrictive amendments offered by Representative William Dannemeyer (R-CA) and Senator Jesse Helms (R-NC), respectively. The conference report was adopted by both houses on August 4, 1990. The final version of the bill authorized $875 million in fiscal 1991 and was signed into law by President Bush on August 18th (*Congressional Quarterly Almanac*, 1990).

As passed, the Ryan White Act provides emergency relief grants to cities with more than 2,000 reported cases of AIDS, HIV-care grants to states to provide health and support services to HIV+ individuals, and funding for early intervention services for persons who have contracted or are at risk to contract HIV. The act specifies that fifteen percent of the HIV-care grants are to be set aside to provide services to infants, children, women, and families with AIDS and up to 10 percent of the grants are to be spent on special projects such as delivering services to hemophiliacs or Native Americans with AIDS. These set-asides are not congruent with the number of PWAs in these target populations. The final version of the law also contained provisions requiring states to develop programs to notify the sexual partners of persons testing HIV+, prohibited the use of federal funds to provide clean needles to injection drug users, and required states to adopt laws criminalizing the intentional transmission of HIV. Funds were authorized to pay for the mandatory testing of prisoners convicted of sex-related crimes, demonstration projects to improve treatment and services to infants and children with AIDS, a study of AIDS in rural areas, and grants to implement emergency-worker guidelines designed to reduce the risk of on-the-job HIV infection.

The Senate floor debate on the Ryan White Act highlights the differentiation of PWA target populations that occurred on both sides of the aisle. Senator David Pryor (D-AK) seems to distinguish the deserving PWAs from those who might not be as deserving—"(PWAs) are not necessarily homosexuals. . . .They are children whose only sin is to be born" (U.S. Congress, Senate, 1990a: S6193). Presumably adults with AIDS are guilty of other sins. Despite the fact that the vast majority of the reported AIDS cases in 1990 were among gays and IDUs, Jesse Helms argued that the act should be focused on more deserving, dependent populations:

> My point is that this legislation should focus on the 2 percent [of PWAs] like Ryan White and like that young woman surgeon from Puerto Rico [who received a tainted blood transfusion]. It should focus on the women and children. (U.S. Congress, Senate, 1990a: S6197)

While the act as passed ultimately distributed the bulk of its funding to states to use for undifferentiated spending on PWAs, it did contain a mix of provisions targeted at specific PWA target populations.

Under the act, deviant PWAs are the subject of policy burdens. Prisoners convicted of sex-related crimes are required to undergo mandatory HIV testing (though no treatment or care funds were targeted at prisoners), IDUs are prohibited from being given clean needles, and the knowing *possible* transmission of HIV becomes a crime. Each of these coercive provisions is a watereddown version of much stricter sanctions: the original proposal for prisoner testing calling for the mandatory testing of all prisoners regardless of crime, an amendment to ban even the distribution of bleach to IDUs in order to allow them to clean their needles and syringes was proposed, and the initial amendment to criminalize the possible transmission of HIV specifically targeted drug users and prostitutes regardless of their HIV status. This later amendment introduced by Senator Helms would have made it a crime to donate blood if an individual:

> who, on or after January 1, 1977 is or has been a user of any intravenous drug . . . (or) has engaged in prostitution. . . . Transmission of the Human Immunodeficiency Virus *does not have to occur* for a person to have committed a violation of this section. (U.S. Congress, Senate, 1990b: S6294, emphasis added)

This amendment would have penalized individuals based solely on their affiliation with a deviant group rather than on their transmission of HIV, as under this language an HIV– person could be convicted.

This amendment was introduced by Helms as the "Ryan White Amendment" and is a good example of a policy being crafted to seemingly provide a generalized benefit (a safe blood supply) and burdens to deviants. It was narrowly defeated (47–52), but what is most interesting is that the rationales offered by opponents of the amendment had little to do with the merits of the amendment as a public health measure. The reasoning most commonly asserted in opposition to the amendment is that it might incorrectly assign rehabilitated "normalized" individuals to a deviant population. Senator Kennedy contended that the amendment would penalize people "who are now completely reformed," while Senator Carl Levin (D-MI) echoed this logic noting that an individual who "successfully underwent drug rehabilitation" could be labeled a criminal if the Helms amendment passed (U.S. Congress, Senate, 1990b: S6301, 6304). As the social construction perspective suggests, there was no disagreement that deviants should be the target of sanctions, only disagreement as to how to properly identify members of those populations in order to maintain the boundaries separating the deserving from undeserving. Under the act, small special project grants were established to improve drug treatment programs but given the burdens placed on IDUs elsewhere in the act, these treatment grants are largely symbolic and serve to bolster the opinions expressed above that IDUs can and should be rehabilitated and reformed. The extension of symbolic grants reinforces the prevailing social construction of IDUs as deviants whose personal culpability now may be viewed as including the failure to take advantage of government assistance.

Deviants were not the only set of target populations differentiated under the Ryan White Act; dependents found themselves designated the recipients of some symbolic and substantive policy benefits. Although nearly 90 percent of the AIDS cases reported through 1990 were among adult men, the Ryan White Act required that 15 percent of the Title II, HIV-care grants be set aside for women and children. This disproportionate funding was justified on the grounds that pediatric AIDS was more expensive than adult AIDS, and that these two populations represented some of the fastest growing segments of the AIDS epidemic. Yet this rationale willfully ignores the previous failures to provide funding for IDUs and inner-city blacks and Hispanics who represent a huge, growing population with AIDS. The deviance of IDUs explains their neglect and the lack of political power possessed by inner-city PWAs probably accounts for the absence of set-asides for that population. In contrast, advocates for children with AIDS are relatively well funded and well organized. Their concerns are represented to Congress by groups such as the Pediatric AIDS Foundation, the Pediatric AIDS Coalition, and the National Hemophilia Foundation. Though ostensibly advocates for all children with AIDS, the children most often the subject of Congressional attention have been "the children with hemophilia or children who have received transfusions, not the children of heroin-injecting minority mothers" (National Research Council, 1993: 211). The clout and the positive construction of this dependent population is witnessed by the fact that of the 17 Congressional hearings on AIDS that took place in the three years leading up to the passage of the Ryan White Act, four (24%) focused exclusively on pediatric AIDS. None of the hearings focused similarly on IDUs and only two centered on the problems of AIDS in the inner city.

This inordinate focus on children with AIDS can be seen as a reflection of the character of public concern for PWAs and/or a strategic emphasis by legislators. Public officials do not simply react to social constructions floating in the ether, but often seek to privilege certain constructions in order to achieve political and policy goals. Despite the women and children set-aside, the majority of the care and treatment funds authorized under the act would ultimately be translated into services delivered to gay men who in 1990 comprised more than half of the documented cases of AIDS. Unlike spending for AIDS research, which allocates funds to a positively constructed biomedical research establishment and, in the best case, produces results that are long lasting and widely dispersed, care and treatment funds are consumed by PWAs. Fearful of the electoral consequences of conferring benefits on a negatively constructed population, yet mindful of the scope of the epidemic and the inability to rationally sustain a policy that would provide treatment for women and children but not for gays, supporters of the act focused on the benefits targeted at positively constructed groups and downplayed the obvious benefits to be received by negatively constructed populations.

The extent to which lawmakers relied on rhetoric to sharpen and solidify the positive construction of children with AIDS is illustrated in the House Select Committee on Children, Youth, and Families' hearing, "AIDS and Young Children in Florida," held the year before passage of the Ryan White Act. Throughout the hearing, the four congressmen present repeatedly spoke of children with AIDS as "innocent" and as "victims." In all, the representatives used the words more than a dozen times. In contrast, none of the nine witnesses ever used these adjectives to describe children with AIDS (U.S. Congress, House, 1989). Perhaps this is a strategy on the part of the witnesses to move the social construction of PWAs away from the innocent/guilty dichotomy. In any event, the use of the rhetoric by the congressmen is not accidental and indicates a clear intention—strategic or not—to portray children with AIDS as a deserving population.

The House and Senate floor debate over the act provides another indication of the attempt to downplay the receipt of benefits by gays while emphasizing the benefits granted to positively constructed populations, most notably children. During the floor debate, lawmakers often relied on stories about PWAs to justify their position on the bill. Supporters of the bill told a total of nineteen such stories. Six members of Congress recounted the story of Ryan White, five told stories focusing on infants or children, three spoke of women, and two spoke of recipients of blood transfusions. Only one story included a protagonist who was identified as being gay or an IDU (both, in this case), and only one story did not reveal the context of HIV infection. This final story, though, recounted the suicide of a distraught man with AIDS who left behind a family, so the sexual identity of the PWA is implicitly heterosexual. These stories are obviously not representative of the demographics of the AIDS epidemic; rather, what they reveal is the intention of policymakers to strongly emphasize the need for the distribution of benefits to positively constructed target populations.

The most obvious example of this strategy to emphasize the distribution of benefits to positively constructed groups was the naming of the bill after the late Ryan White. Ryan White's death in April 1990 was widely reported in both print and electronic media and he was eulogized in each of the three major news magazines. Attaching such a potent symbol to the bill allowed its supporters to easily communicate to the public their preferred spin on legislation. Opponents of the bill understood this as well. Senator Helms saw the bill as a Trojan horse delivering benefits to gay PWAs under the guise of services to women and children. He made his feelings known: ". . . you better believe that the so-called homosexual community understood that Ryan White's story was just too good to pass up, too great an opportunity" (U.S. Congress, Senate 1990a, S6195).

While supporters of the act never mentioned the gay lobby during debate on the bill, after the bill was passed gay rights organizations hailed the law as a victory and stressed how instrumental their support for the bill had been (Castaneda, 1990). This is an excellent example of the quiet delivery of benefits to a negatively constructed target population, justified by rationales that stressed the benefits to be conferred on positively constructed populations. This interpretation is further supported by the fact that the initial draft of the bill contained a provision allowing states to waive the women and children set-asides. During debate over the bill the waiver provision was deleted; however, as originally conceived, the major substantive benefit targeted at women and children was largely symbolic.

In sum, the battle over the Ryan White CARE Act can be seen as a battle over which social constructions of the epidemic and which people affected by the epidemic would be privileged. Supporters of the bill succeeded in crafting a version of the epidemic that emphasized its women and children "victims" and deemphasized the extent to which benefits would be delivered to negatively constructed groups. This strategy was made possible by an expansion in the social understanding of who is at risk for HIV/AIDS, which can be traced to the 1985 Hudson/White media event. Societal learning about AIDS and the construction of multiple categories of PWAs has certainly served to direct burdens at deviant groups, but, as illustrated above, such a fluid construction also presented a means for lawmakers to deliver benefits to a negatively constructed target population while maintaining the apparent congruence between social constructions and policy outputs in the eyes of the public.

LESSONS FROM AIDS

AIDS policies can be understood by looking at the ways in which different groups of people with AIDS have been socially constructed. The design of policy—often, as observers point out, a policy of inaction—can be attributed in some important ways to the manner in which different groups of PWAs have been constructed in the eyes of the public and federal policymakers. The Ryan White Act, with its punitive policies toward injection drug users and its special set-aside provisions for women and children with AIDS, highlights this point. The failure of Congress to fund the act's provisions at the authorized levels—only eighteen percent ($159 million) of the amount authorized was appropriated in 1990 and the act has yet to be fully funded—indicates that, despite the emergence of positively constructed groups of PWAs, people with AIDS still have relatively little political power.

The narrative presented here should be familiar to anyone well acquainted with the history of HIV/AIDS in the United States. The social construction perspective, though, provides a means for systematically discussing important issues that have long been a part of the debate about AIDS policy. When policies differentiate between different groups of citizens in order to target benefits and burdens at them—and this is almost always the case with social policies—a social construction perspective that identifies and examines the role of group stereotypes must be a central part of the analysis. To make such a perspective even more useful, I close with three propositions that crystallize the lessons of this chapter and can hopefully be generalized beyond the important case of AIDS.

Target populations are constructed using meanings derived from three key sources: (1) historical categories affiliated with episodic policy problems, (2) technical definitions and categories created by professionals and experts in a given policy domain, and (3) cultural stereotypes of groups objectively associated with the policy problem.

This first proposition attempts to formalize an answer to the very basic question: Where do target populations come from? The sources of meaning used to construct target populations are threefold. First, problem definitions often carry presumptions about the relevant target populations. The appearance of AIDS resulted in an initial categorization of target populations that seems to have had more to do with familiar historical responses to epidemics (distinguishing, for example, between "victims" and "carriers") than it did the intrinsic properties of the public policy dilemmas posed by the epidemic. These categories were not medical categories employed because of the similarities between HIV/AIDS and previous epidemics, rather, the categories that drove policy were historically imbedded ones that were, in fact, at odds with the scientific understanding of the epidemic. The mechanism through which a historically scripted set of categories is created is unclear. I would speculate that certain events—plagues in this case—are of such a magnitude and generate so much fear that a social memory develops that is recalled when similar events recur.

In addition to historically generated categories of target populations, professional groups confronting a policy problem bring their own routine categories and technical definitions to bear on the problem. People with AIDS may be seen by doctors as patients suffering from an STD or by medical researchers as subjects for clinical drug trials. This second source of target population construction has influence on the design of policy, but because the categories are generated by specialized communities they will be vulnerable to wider political forces when the issue becomes a "policy with a public" and is the subject of widespread media coverage and public discussion (May, 1991).

The social construction of target populations is also centrally related to the context of a policy problem. The AIDS epidemic spawned target populations centered initially around homosexual sexual behavior and drug use, which in turn unleashed existing cultural stereotypes and affective responses to these groups. This set of target populations certainly would not have been constructed had HIV been spread by an insect vector (such as mosquitoes), as is the case with malaria. As policymakers and political activists attempt to construct target populations that will further their goals, they draw on the meanings provided by historical, technical, and cultural categories. In a given policy area, each of these sources may exist simultaneously, and the manipulation and interaction of these different categories is an important factor leading to changes in the social construction of target populations over time.

When public events are incongruous with the existing construction of target populations, new target populations will be constructed.

As perceptions of a policy problem change over time, often the construction of target populations will change as well. If a problem is viewed as afflicting (or being caused by) people not already included in a target population, then the underlying causal theory connecting the policy problem to the target population is threatened and a degree of social dissonance arises. Three responses are possible: (1) the evidence can be ignored and the causal theory left intact (heterosexuals do not get AIDS, therefore those with AIDS must really be gay), (2) additional target populations can be constructed and the causal theory amended (gays get AIDS, but so do women and children— for different reasons), or (3) existing definitions of target populations can be modified along with the causal theory (being a member of a group does not determine your risk for AIDS, engaging in certain behavior does).

In the case of HIV/AIDS, evidence that the threat of HIV infection is more widespread than initially believed has slowly worked its way through the first two possible responses. Initially there was widespread public denial that certain groups—heterosexuals in particular—were at risk for AIDS despite medical evidence to the contrary. This gave way to the second response in the face of Rock Hudson's announcement and the publicizing of the Ryan White case. It is more likely that policy dissonance will be dealt with by adding a new target population than by altering the affective response to an already existing one. In many ways passage of the Ryan White Act was facilitated by the addition of new, ostensibly more deserving categories of people with AIDS. Before this shift lawmakers did not perceive the extension of benefits to PWAs as defensible in light of the prevailing image of AIDS sufferers. Throughout most of the epidemic many medical professionals and AIDS activists have steadily pushed for the third response, which would result in medicalizing the discussion of people with AIDS and ceasing to distinguish the deservedness of infected persons based on the mode of HIV transmission. However, the continued marginalization of many groups of people with AIDS indicates that this understanding of HIV/AIDS has not yet been widely adopted outside of some medical and activist circles.

Though different target populations may be subjected to similar risks, the policies directed at these populations will often vary depending on the perceived deservedness of each group.

While this proposition is implicit in Schneider and Ingram's work, making it explicit highlights the way in which social constructions may serve as barriers to efficient and equitable policymaking, particularly where problems and the relationship between different target populations are complex. This is starkly demonstrated by the difference in policies targeted at injection drug users and children with AIDS. Lawmakers have shown considerably more concern for the plight of infected children than they have for infected IDUs and the effect of this concern on the design of policy is illustrated in the way in which each group is treated under the Ryan White Act. The fact that varied social constructions spawn varied policies is a matter of substantive concern. The prevalent sense that injection drug users are deviant and undeserving hinders public health efforts to stem the epidemic among this group and has led to increasing rates of HIV infection among their sexual partners and children. In 1985, 73 percent of the cases of heterosexual transmission of HIV and 51 percent of the pediatric cases documented by the CDC were traceable to injection drug users (DesJarlais, Friedman, & Hopkins,1988). Quite clearly, the construction of injection drug users as undeserving has had the unintended consequence of inhibiting efforts to reduce the rates of infection among ostensibly more deserving populations. When social constructions of target populations drive policymaking, the result can be inefficient and inequitable policy solutions that serve to severely undermine the social intelligence of responses to serious policy problems.

REFERENCES

Altman, D. (1986). *AIDS in the Mind of America.* New York: Anchor Press/Doubleday.

Bayer, R. (1989). *Private Acts, Social Consequences: AIDS and the Politics of Public Health.* New York: The Free Press.

Brandt, A. M. (1985). *No Magic Bullet: A Social History of Venereal Disease in the United States Since 1880.* New York: Oxford University Press.

Brandt, A. M. (1988). AIDS: From social history to social policy, in Fee, E., & D. M. Fox, eds. *AIDS: The Burdens of History,* 147-71. Berkeley: University of California Press.

Castaneda, R. (1990). Gay rights fund-raiser marks gains; Group cites 3 progressive bills, ties with hill, White House. *Washington Post,* 7 October, B3 (Metro). Lexis text retrieval.

Centers for Disease Control and Prevention. (1994). *HIV/AIDS Surveillance Report*, 6:1.

——. (1993). AIDS information: Statistical projections and trends, fax information service document # 320210 (January 1st).

Cook, T. E., & D. C. Colby. (1992). The mass-mediated epidemic, in Fee, E., & D. M. Fox, eds. *AIDS: The Making of a Chronic Disease*, 84–122. Berkeley: University of California Press.

Corea, G. (1992). *The Invisible Epidemic: The Story of Women and AIDS*. New York: Harper-Collins.

Congressional Quarterly Almanac. (1990). Washington D.C.: Congressional Quarterly, Inc.

Crimp, D., ed. (1987). *AIDS: Cultural Analysis/Cultural Activism.* Boston: MIT Press.

Dearing, J. W. (1992). Foreign blood and domestic politics. In Fee, E., & D. M. Fox, eds. *AIDS: The Making of a Chronic Disease*, 326–45. Berkeley: University of California Press.

DesJarlais, D. C., N. Jainchill, & S. R. Friedman. (1988). AIDS among IV drug users: Epidemiology, natural history, and therapeutic community experiences, in Galea R., Lewis B., & Baker L., eds. *AIDS and IV Drug Users*, 51–59. Owings Mill, MD: National Health Publishing.

Epstein, S. (1991). Democratic science? AIDS activism and the contested construction of knowledge. *Socialist Review*, 21(April-June): 35–64.

Fee, E. (1988). Sin versus science: venereal disease in twentieth-century Baltimore, in Fee E., & Fox, D. M., eds. *AIDS: The Burdens of History.*, 121–46. Berkeley: University of California Press.

Fox, D. (1992). The politics of HIV infection: 1989–1990 as years of change, in Fee, E., & Fox, D. M., eds. *AIDS: The Making of a Chronic Disease*, 125–43. Berkeley: University of California Press.

Gilman, S. L. (1988). *Disease and Representation: Images of Illness from Madness to AIDS.* Ithaca: Cornell University Press.

Grmek, M. D. (1990). *History of AIDS: Emergence and Origin of a Modern Pandemic.* (R. C. Maulitz & J. Duffin, trans.). Princeton: Princeton University Press.

Hombs, M. E. (1992). *AIDS Crisis in America.* Santa Barbara, CA: ABC-CLIO. *Journal of Policy Analysis and Management*, 12 (Summer): 438–55.

Hughes, C. G. (1993). The piper's dance: a paradigm of the collective response to epidemic disease. *International Journal of Mass Emergencies and Disasters*, 11(August): 227–45.

Hughey, J. D., R. W. Norton & C. Sullivan-Norton. (1989). Insidious metaphors and the changing meaning of AIDS. *AIDS & Public Policy Journal*, 4(Spring): 56–67.

Kinsella, J. (1989). *Covering the Plague: AIDS and the American Media.* New Brunswick: Rutgers University Press.

Kirp, D. L. & R. Bayer. (1992). The second decade of AIDS: The end to exceptionalism? in Kirp, D. L., & Bayer, R., eds. *AIDS in the Industrialized Democracies*, 361–84. New Brunswick: Rutgers University Press.

Kirp, D. L., with S. Epstein, et al. (1989). *Learning by Heart: AIDS and Schoolchildren in America's Communities.* New Brunswick: Rutgers University Press.

Mack, A., ed. (1991). *In Time of Plague: The History and Social Consequences of Lethal Epidemic Disease.* New York: New York University Press.

MacKinnon, K. (1992). *The Politics of Popular Representation: Reagan, Thatcher, AIDS, and the Movies.* Cranbury, NJ: Associated University Press.

May, P. J. (1991). Reconsidering policy design: Policies and publics. *Journal of Public Policy*, 11 (Part 2): 287–306.

Meredith, A. (1992). Until that last breath: Women with AIDS, in Fee, E., & D. M. Fox, eds. *AIDS: The Making of a Chronic Disease*, 229–44. Berkeley: University of California Press.

Misztal, B., & D. Moss, eds. (1990). *Action on AIDS: National Policies in Comparative Perspective.* New York: Greenwood Press.

National Research Council. (1993). *The Social Impact of AIDS in the United States.* Washington, D.C.: National Academy Press.

———. (1990). *AIDS: The Second Decade.* Washington, D.C.: National Academy Press.

Nelkin, D., & S. L. Gilman. (1991). Placing blame for devastating disease, in Mack A., ed. *In Time of Plague: The History and Social Consequences of Lethal Epidemic Disease,* 39–56. New York: New York University Press.

Perrow, C., & M. F. Guillén. (1990). *The AIDS Disaster: The Failure of Organizations in New York and the Nation.* New Haven: Yale University Press.

Presidential Commission on the Human Immunodeficiency Virus Epidemic. (1988). *Report of the Presidential Commission on the Human Immunodeficiency Virus Epidemic.* Washington, D.C.: Government Printing Office.

Price, C. (1992). AIDS, organization of drug users, and public policy. *AIDS & Public Policy Journal,* 7(Fall): 141–44.

Quam, M., & N. Ford. (1990). AIDS policies and practices in the United States, in Misztal B., & Moss D., eds. *Action on AIDS: National Policies in Comparative Perspective,* 25–50. New York: Greenwood Press.

Rogers, E. M., J. W. Dearing, & S. Chang. (1991). AIDS in the 1980s: The agenda-setting process for a public issue. *Journalism Monographs,* No. 126. Association for Education in Journalism and Mass Communication.

Ron, A., & D. E. Rogers. (1989). AIDS in the United States: Patient care and politics. *Daedalus,* 118:2 (Spring): 41–58.

Rosenberg, C. (1989). What is an epidemic? AIDS in historical perspective. *Daedalus,* 118:2 (Spring): 1–17.

Ryan White Comprehensive AIDS Resources Emergency Act of 1990. (1990). *U.S. code* (P.L. 101–381).

Schneider, A., & H. Ingram. (1993). The social construction of target populations: Implications for politics and policy. *American Political Science Review,* 87(June): 334–47.

Shilts, R. (1987). *And the Band Played on: Politics, People, and the AIDS Epidemic.* New York: Penguin Books.

Treichler, P. A. (1988). AIDS, gender, and biomedical discourse, in Fee, E., & Fox, D. M., eds. *AIDS: The Burdens of History.* 190–266. Berkeley: University of California Press.

U.S. Congress. House. (1989). Select Committee on Children, Youth, and Families. *AIDS and Young Children in South Florida.* 101st Cong., 1st Sess., 7 August.

U.S. Congress. Senate. (1990a). 101st Cong., 2nd Sess. *Congressional Record* (15 May), vol. 136, pt. 1.

———. ———. (1990b). 101st Cong., 2nd Sess. *Congressional Record* (16 May), vol. 136, pt. 1.

Wachter, R. M. (1992). AIDS, activism, and the politics of health. *The New England Journal of Medicine,* (January 9th): 128–33.

7

AIDS: Perspectives on Public Health, Policy, and Administration

James A. Johnson and Walter J. Jones

As in other areas of administration, the uncertainties and contingencies of federalism that underlie the American system of public health management are most sharply brought into focus during periods of crisis. During these times, there are usually important gaps in the factual knowledge necessary for administrators to act. In addition, there is often political conflict over both the definition of the crisis and the governmental actions necessary to address it. If strong national leadership does not exist, or is not predisposed to expend political capital to bring about coherent national policy, the action drifts to the states and localities, which will feature almost every variation between robust activism and complete inactivity. The danger is, of course, that this pattern of activity may not be enough to ward off an ever-expanding disaster.

In public health, no crisis has loomed more ominously over the heads of administrators in the last several decades than the ongoing epidemic of Acquired Immune Deficiency Syndrome (AIDS). It first attracted the attention of public health workers in a handful of cities (in particular, San Francisco, New York, Miami, and Los Angeles) in the early eighties. Since then, the disease has expanded geographically to cover all major cities and, increasingly, rural areas as well. AIDS infection is now also increasingly spreading

Johnson, James A. and Jones, Walter J. From "AIDS: Perspectives on Public Health, Policy, and Administration," *Public Administration Review* (September/October 1991), pp. 456–60. Reprinted by permission from Public Administration Review © by the American Society for Public Administration (ASPA), 1120 G Street, Suite 700, Washington, DC 20005. All rights reserved.

from its initial concentrations in gay and IV–drug using groups to other seg-ments of the population, including sexually active heterosexuals in all age groups (Centers for Disease Control, 1991).

However, research into the specific functioning of the HIV virus leading to AIDS is still incomplete. It is unlikely that an AIDS vaccine will be available during the 1990s. An additional public health obstacle is that the activities most likely to lead to AIDS transmission—unprotected sex and needle shar-ing—are highly resistant to modification through education or legal sanction (Bayer, 1989).

The reaction of public health administrators to the growing AIDS threat has been quite varied—surprisingly so, given the professional consen-sus on the seriousness of the epidemic. As in other policy areas, the federal government has in the last decade been inclined to view public health administration as an area more properly left to the states and localities (Williams and Torrens, 1988). More particularly, in the case of AIDS, admin-istrators concerned with education and health in the Reagan and Bush administrations have been ideologically divided on the proper response, with those placing primary emphasis on education to minimize the risks of sex and drug use pitted against other administrators who favor a more puni-tive and sanctions-oriented approach that is supposed to reduce or elimi-nate risky activities altogether (Jones and Johnson, 1988). Given the federal budgetary situation, few if any national policymakers wish to confront the issue of long-term care for the large number of people with AIDS who will need it in the coming years. The primary result of this impasse has been that the federal Executive Branch has largely limited itself to funding AIDS research and left more practical AIDS education, prevention, and treatment to the states and localities, as well as individual public and private sector organizations. It is true that the federal courts in landmark decisions such as *Arline v. Nassau County* have provided national parameters on legally accept-able policies.

Additionally, health care facilities have undeniably been subjected to progressively more detailed regulations from Occupational Safety and Health Administration (OSHA) and the Centers for Disease Control (CDC) regard-ing such matters as the application of "universal precautions" in situations involving the potential transmission of bodily fluids (Wilson and Elliot, 1989; Jones and Johnson, 1989). Nevertheless, the states and localities have, if only by default, preserved a wide latitude on what can or should be done.

Any analysis of how well public health administration is coping with the AIDS epidemic must begin with the *Morbidity and Mortality Weekly Report (MMWR)* (1991). This weekly report tracks trends and developments in dis-ease control and provides the most current and comprehensive data on the spread of human immunodeficiency virus (HIV) in the U.S. From 1981 through 1990, 100,777 deaths among persons with AIDS were reported to CDC by local, state, and territorial health departments; almost one third of these deaths were reported during 1990. During the 1980s, AIDS emerged as a leading cause of death among young adults in the United States. By 1989, HIV infection/AIDS had surpassed heart disease, cancer, suicide, and homicide to become the second leading cause of death among men 25–44 years of age. Based on current trends, HIV infection/AIDS is likely to rank among the five leading causes of death among women 25–44 years of age in 1991.

According to the *MMWR*, most deaths from AIDS have occurred among homosexual and bisexual men (59 percent) and among women and heterosexual men who are intravenous-drug users (21 percent). Nearly three fourths of the deaths occurred among persons 25–44 years of age. Although most deaths occurred among whites, death rates have been highest for blacks and Hispanics. During 1990, the number of reported deaths per 100,000 population was 29.3 for blacks, 22.2 for Hispanics, 8.7 for whites, 2.8 for Asian/Pacific Islanders, and 2.8 for American Indians/Alaskan Natives.

The impact of HIV infection/AIDS on mortality in the mid-1990s to late 1990s and early 2000s will depend on present efforts to prevent and treat HIV infection, and on how the characteristics of the epidemic—and social responses to it—evolve in the years to come. For example, in San Francisco, Los Angeles, and New York City, AIDS is the leading cause of death among young adult men. In both New York State and New Jersey, AIDS is the leading cause of death among black women 15–44 years of age; in New Jersey, the number of deaths among this population from AIDS in 1988 was nearly equal to the number of deaths from the second and third leading causes combined (cancer and unintentional injuries). In some locations, AIDS has become a major cause of death among young children; in New York State in 1988, AIDS was the leading cause of death among Hispanic children 1–4 years of age, and the second leading cause of death among black children 1–4 years of age, exceeding deaths from unintentional injuries among Hispanic children and from all other infectious diseases among both groups.

In addition to mortality statistics, measures of the public health impact of AIDS include morbidity, disability, and health care costs. For example, the AIDS epidemic is straining the resources of public hospitals; in 1989, private insurers paid more than an estimated one billion dollars for reimbursement of AIDS–related claims for life and health insurance, an increase of 71 percent from 1988.

An estimated one million persons in the United States are infected with HIV; of these, an estimated 165,000–215,000 will die during 1991–1993. The impact of HIV infection/AIDS on mortality in the mid–1990s to late 1990s and early 2000s will depend on present efforts to prevent and treat HIV infection.

In an effort to understand these issues, *AIDS: The Second Decade* (1990) was prepared by the Committee on AIDS Research and the Behavioral, Social, and Statistical Sciences, which was established in 1987. The formation of such a committee within the National Research Council reflected a growing awareness that understanding HIV transmission, facilitating behavioral change to prevent further spread of infection, and coping with the social consequences of the epidemic raise questions that properly lie within the domain of the social, behavioral, and statistical sciences. At the request of the Public Health Service (PHS) and with support from the Russell Sage and Rockefeller Foundations, the committee reviewed estimates of the extent of HIV infection in the U.S. population and the patterns of sexual behavior and drug use that transmit HIV. It also reviewed intervention strategies that showed promise of producing behavioral change to slow the spread of HIV infection in the general population.

With this report, the committee continues the work it began in 1987 to monitor the AIDS epidemic and to investigate issues related to preventing the transmission of HIV. The topics addressed in the report span a range of substantive areas, from improving the quality of survey data on behaviors associated with HIV transmission to modifying the behavior of blood donors.

In the second decade of the epidemic, as indicated in the report, new pockets of infection are being identified in more diverse geographical locations in the United States, and the changing distributions of AIDS cases and HIV infection indicate that the disease is becoming more a generalized American phenomenon and less a bicoastal, urban entity. Moreover, the pattern of infection is beginning to reveal some subtle shifts in the distribution of AIDS cases across transmission categories; the proportion of cases attributable to same-gender contact has decreased slightly as the proportion ascribed to heterosexual contact has grown. Even the characteristics of the disease itself are somewhat in flux. With the development of drugs capable of decreasing morbidity associated with HIV infection and prolonging the lives of those infected with the virus, the disease takes on some of the characteristics of a long-term rather than an acute illness. The changing locus of the epidemic, the new populations at risk, and the emerging longer term nature of the disease point to the need for new outreach and intervention strategies to prevent further spread of infection, as well as services and treatment to assist those who are already infected.

After a decade of struggle against AIDS, the central question raised in the report is: Where do we go from here? Some individuals claim that the epidemic has peaked and no longer needs the attention—and resources—that have been directed toward it in the past. Others say that there are more pressing problems facing our nation. The committee, although recognizing the frustration that often underlies such viewpoints, finds little credible evidence that the end of this epidemic is in sight. As stated, the picture for the near future is one of a continuing toll of sickness and death. Behavioral change continues to be the primary weapon in retarding the spread of HIV. Amassing the knowledge needed to better understand and facilitate behavioral change will require a long-term commitment to rigorous scientific investigation.

As suggested earlier, however, present-day public health responses to AIDS are primarily at the state and local level. One interesting example of what a local government can do to come to grips with AIDS is shown in *Responding to the Growing Challenge of AIDS in Shelby County, Tennessee* (1989). Shelby County is the most populous county in the state of Tennessee, containing over one million residents. In addition, it is demographically quite diverse, containing a major city (Memphis), with a large black population, along with numerous small towns and rural communities. Wide variations in education, income, and social behavior also exist.

Faced with a rapidly increasing AIDS caseload, Shelby County governmental and public health agencies formed an Advisory Committee to devise proper responses. The recommendations of the Advisory Committee are grounded in the belief that an adequate response by the community to the challenge of AIDS must encompass the following objectives: (1) to ensure that persons with HIV–related illness receive adequate medical, health care, and social services; (2) to prevent the spread of HIV infection to uninfected members of the community; (3) to protect persons with HIV infection from discrimination and other violations of their legal rights; and (4) to provide services to HIV–infected persons in a manner that will cause the least disruption in the ability of county officials to continue services essential to the welfare of the community.

These considerations suggest the key features outlined in this report that must be possessed by an adequate system of health care and social services. First, the system must include a variety of different types of services, including medical, mental health, home health care, dental, and social services. Second, the system must include various levels of health care services, delivered in the ambulatory clinic, hospital, and home, as appropriate. Third, there must be effective management and coordination of services for each patient, thereby ensuring ready access to all necessary services in the least disruptive and least costly setting possible.

The system of health care and social services described for persons with AIDS must include several components described in the advisory report. Ambulatory care is the cornerstone of the system. It would ideally incorporate a number of services, including "day hospital care" (including I.V. therapy), mental health services, dental care, rehabilitation programs, nutritional counseling, and clinical laboratory and radiology services. Primary care in this setting would be provided by internists and family practitioners, with ready access to a variety of specialists. Ambulatory care might be provided in doctors' offices, clinics, or special centers.

Home health care services must be developed that permit persons with AIDS to remain in their own homes rather than being institutionalized in hospitals or nursing homes. Home services should include assistance in activities of daily living, psychological counseling, and routine nursing care.

In addition, there is a growing need for group residences, serving person in the late stages of their illness who need specialized care and are unable to remain living at home. These facilities would provide attendant care and access to services of a multidisciplinary team of health care workers. While these facilities would function like the traditional hospice in providing rigorous supportive care, they would not exclude persons with AIDS who continue to undergo aggressive therapy for life-threatening complications of their disease. Nursing homes offering intermediate and skilled levels of nursing care might also fulfill a portion of the need in this area. Although it was not possible to survey local nursing homes, it is believed that few, if any, are willing to accept AIDS patients. Lack of access to long-term care facilities represents a serious gap in the system of services for persons with AIDS.

Social service agencies need to locate offices in close proximity to sites where persons with AIDS receive health care. This will facilitate their efforts to receive financial assistance and other services (such as Social Security and Medicaid benefits). These services are especially important, since most persons with AIDS exhaust personal resources in the course of their illness.

Finally, a mechanism for case management and coordination of care for person with AIDS is essential to the effective administration of the health care and social services system. The basic function of case managers would be to assist persons with AIDS in identifying and gaining access to needed services and to encourage the provision of health care in the least disruptive and costly settings. These case managers must be professionals fully knowledgeable about the array of available services. They must be available to interact regularly and on a personal basis with their clients. They must also have access to the medical, psychosocial, and financial data about patients that will enable them to provide effective counsel and assistance.

The *AIDS Prevention and Services Workshop* (1990) was designed to disseminate information that could be used by governments to move toward such a system. Conducted by the National Health Policy Forum through a grant for the Robert Wood Johnson Foundation, the workshop brought together selected foundation grantees. The National Health Policy Forum is a nonpartisan education and information exchange for senior federal health policymakers, including White House and congressional staff and others in the many agencies responsible for health programs and delivery. Guided by a steering committee of key congressional and regulatory health officials, it has served for more than 18 years to provide frequent contact with leaders from the corporate, provider, and research communities.

The Robert Wood Johnson Foundation so far has been the principal source of private funds to provide preventive and health services for people with AIDS and HIV infection. The purpose of the conference was to provide an opportunity for some of the foundation's AIDS grantees to share what they have learned. Their primary conclusion is that American public policy has failed in a number of areas. To begin with, after 10 years, there is great difficulty in predicting how many people are being infected with HIV daily. Therefore, the public health community has no way of making a rational response or developing an appropriate strategy.

Second, for years there has been discussion about the need for financial restructuring, for housing, and for collateral services, and adequate action has still not been taken. In the meantime, hundreds of thousands of people have been infected and need services. The big metropolitan areas have provided a glimpse of what the whole nation could face in the future with the biggest increases in areas that have not yet been hit with HIV.

Third, there appears to be a bureaucratic maze. The leadership vacuum for HIV and AIDS policy has left the nation with budget analysts who have no public-policy training to make program and policy decisions. The assistant commissioner of AIDS Prevention and Control for New Jersey shared a story in which a financial analyst said to him, in regard to the New Jersey Treatment Assessment Program, "Well it would be cheaper to let them die, wouldn't it?" Values like these—rather than fairness, justice, and humanity—are being brought into play in making AIDS policy.

Finally—there are issues pertaining to the "decimation of minority and disenfranchised populations by HIV and AIDS." As indicated by the CDC reports, the epidemic is now becoming less associated with risk groups and more related to socioeconomic factors.

Along with the public policy vacuum, the report identifies a crisis in HIV and AIDS care and treatment. The states, and especially the high incidence states, cannot absorb the cost of the care and treatment for this epidemic. The difficulty in AIDS financing is clearly demonstrated in the state of New Jersey. There is an uncompensated care fund of $500 million for all residents who are uninsured or underinsured. Yet the 1992 cost for diagnosed AIDS cases alone is expected to be $1 billion.

As described in the proceedings, AIDS has been addressed by many agencies at the federal level, most under the Department of Health and Human Services. The Food and Drug Administration, the National Institutes of Health, the Centers for Disease Control, the Health Resources and Services Administration, and the Health Care Financing Administration all have different funding responsibilities and interests with regard to AIDS. Direction and strategy for these agencies, individually and collectively, have been limited.

A multi-year look at the Health Resources and Services Administration (HRSA) AIDS budget exemplifies the lack of strategy in the federal approach. Covering more than nine major service areas, the HRSA AIDS budget has more than quadrupled over the past five years. Only two programs have had long-term stable funding—home health services and sub-acute care, two programs first set up in FY 1990, which also expire at the end of FY 1990. As a result, there is no request for funding these programs in FY 1991, and no planning for their continuation. Funding levels currently approved by Congress will not meet HRSA operating costs for commitments already in place to 25 sites participating in service demonstration projects. And, while housing needs are severe for people with AIDS, HRSA's facilities' renovation program stems from legislation developed for hospitals; thus a costly and possibly unnecessary medical component must accompany housing program plans considered for support under this revenue source.

It is obvious that AIDS service delivery planning must be improved if the unique needs of patients are to be met within the stringent cost limitations currently existing. What are the prospects for such improvements? Not good, according to *Community-Based Care of Persons with AIDS: Developing a Research Agenda* (1990). These proceedings of the Agency for Health Care Policy and Research (AHCPR) conference indicate that health services planning for AIDS depends on highly uncertain projections of future cases and the challenge of assessing health care needs while treatment protocols change rapidly. Federal planning for health services is limited to budget impact analyses; most planning is proceeding at state and local levels. Readiness varies considerably among states and cities. Some areas have no plan while others have a variety of plans assembled by different groups.

According to the report, research on HIV infection, projection methods, and needs assessment tools is needed. Uncertainty about the magnitude of future AIDS incidence and the prevalence of HIV infection is a major problem for planners and policymakers, causing discord and providing an excuse for inactivity. Having little experience with epidemiologic projection models, planners should exercise caution to avoid exaggeration of future need. Policymakers should be careful to avoid the tendency to substitute large-scale planning efforts for the actual provision of needed services.

The report calls for AIDS–related health services research to guide policy and health planning in the allocation of resources and design of health service programs. The following are the pertinent research and policy questions identified:

- What are the current and projected needs, demands, utilization patterns, and costs of the various components of the HIV care continuum?
- What factors affect the reliability and confidence of these projections? How can they be improved?
- What methodologies can be developed to translate data regarding disease patterns and intensity, patient factors, and functional impairment into patient care requirements?
- Can longitudinal studies of cohorts of HIV–infected individuals be developed to identify the ranges of services and resources needed over the duration of the illness?
- How does integration and coordination of provider organizations affect service delivery, accessibility, continuity, quality, and cost of care?
- What are appropriate chronic care outcome measures for the assessment of populations living with HIV illness?

- What would be the impact on the clinical course of HIV infection, cost, and resource utilization (short- and long-term) as a result of the initiation of a national health policy for early treatment of asymptomatic seropositive persons?
- How does the care of AIDS populations compare and vary (cost, resource utilization outcomes) from region to region? Provider to provider? With other chronic illness groups?
- What is the impact on the funding sources for AIDS care ("cost-shifting") of early treatment?

CONCLUSION

An astute observer of health policymaking in the United States recently suggested that the current situation could be best summarized by the saying "if you don't know where you're going, any road will take you" (Sultz, 1991). Since current health policy in general features indecision and serious ideological conflict, it is not surprising that there is still no national consensus on what should be done in the areas of AIDS education, prevention, and treatment.

As the above reports indicate, public health administrators still lack vital information on the ultimate course of the AIDS epidemic. In addition, many of the problems that are resulting from the spread of AIDS, such as the need for long-term care for people with AIDS (PWAs), require coordinated and adequately funded approaches, while the current administrative situation features decentralization and increasingly severe fiscal constraints on state and local as well as federal levels.

Certainly, as observers of current federalism have noted, public administrators have often been able to develop highly innovative and cost-effective responses to problems in spite of such obstacles (Rubin, 1988). The State of New York, among others, has engaged in path-breaking research into the determinants of the AIDS epidemic (Novick, 1991). Numerous local governments have also participated in cooperative efforts at AIDS education, prevention, and treatment (Helgerson, 1984). Without a clear consensus of what should be done, it might even be safer from a public health standpoint (as well as politically wiser) to refrain from a uniform, nationally imposed AIDS policy, and permit state and local administrators to tailor their approaches to the specific needs of their own constituencies.

Such optimism, however, at bottom rests on two articles of faith: that state and local administrators can indeed develop, finance, and implement effective programs to address the varied problems stemming from AIDS with only modest federal assistance, and that the development of the AIDS epidemic will be predictable and gradual enough to let such an incremental and uncoordinated approach work. But AIDS, like any epidemic, spreads without regard to administrative jurisdiction, federal doctrine, or budgetary limitation. Our faith in a decentralized administrative response thus constitutes a gigantic, high stakes gamble. It might even be considered the highest risk behavior of all with respect to the threat of AIDS.

REFERENCES

Bayer, Ronald, 1989. *Private Acts, Social Consequences.* New York, NY: The Free Press, ch. 7.

Helgerson, Stephen, 1984. "AIDS Project in Seattle, Washington." *American Journal of Public Health*, vol. 74 (December), pp. 1419.

Jones, Walter J. and James A. Johnson, 1988. "AIDS: The Urban Policymaking Challenge." *Journal of Urban Affairs*, vol. 11 (March), pp. 85–101.

Jones, Walter J. and James A. Johnson, 1989. "AIDS in the Workplace: Legal and Policy Considerations for Personnel Managers." *Review of Public Personnel Administration*, vol. 9 (Summer), pp. 3–14.

Novick, Lloyd F., ed., 1991. *New York State HIV Seroprevalence Project.* Washington, DC: American Public Health Association.

Rubin, Irene S., 1988. "Municipal Enterprises: Exploring Budgetary and Political Implications." *Public Administration Review*, vol. 48 (January/February), pp. 542–550.

Sultz, Henry, 1991. "If You Don't Know Where You're Going, Any Road Will Take You." *American Journal of Public Health*, vol. 81 (April), pp. 418–420.

Williams, Stephen J. and Paul R. Torrens, eds., 1988. *Introduction to Health Services*, 3d ed. New York: John Wiley & Sons.

Wilson, Thomas and Robert Elliott, 1989. "Legal and Policy Implications." In James A. Johnson, ed., *AIDS in the Workplace.* Memphis, TN: Shelby House, pp. 33–43.

8

Health Care and AIDS

Jonathan Peck and Clement Bezold

Powerfully entrenched forces in the American health care system resist fundamental reform, but the spread of the acquired immune deficiency syndrome (AIDS),[1] combined with other developments, creates new forces for change. Public policy clashes will pit established interests against these new forces. The outcome is unpredictable. Everything about AIDS—from mutations of the virus to society's response—is permeated with enormous uncertainty. Moreover, the politics of health care makes most predictions more an exercise in ideology than forecasting. Nevertheless, we can look at an array of developments that will be triggered or amplified by AIDS and begin to see the dim outlines of a very different health care system that is likely to emerge in the early twenty-first century. . . .

THE CURRENT SYSTEM

The health care system that American public policy helped build provides the most costly health care on the planet. In 1991, the United States spent 12.2 percent of its gross national product on health care, while the average for developed countries was only 7.4 percent.[2] Despite this high amount of

Jonathan Peck and Clement Bezold, "Health Care and AIDS," from *Annals of the American Academy of Political and Social Sciences* (July 1992), pp. 130–139. Reprinted by permission of Sage Publications, Inc.

money spent on health care, there are still well over 30 million Americans who do not have health insurance and thus have limited access to health care. It is often pointed out that no other industrialized nation except South Africa does not have a national health insurance program. It is the uninsured population and Medicaid that will bear the brunt of AIDS infections in the early 1990s.

The international comparisons are made difficult by the fact that the major correlate of ill health, namely, poverty, is not dealt with as well in the United States as in other advanced nations. In effect, we give the poor less effective general assistance, allowing disease to become more prevalent and more intense. Then we often attack the acute stages of disease "with both guns blazing at the symptoms."[3] Thus comparisons of gross outcomes such as life expectancy and infant mortality, which clearly put the United States way behind other developed countries that spend far less of their gross national product for health care, are simplistic.[4] Nonetheless, it is true that, while the U.S. system is the best in the world, at the cutting edge of high technology, it does not serve the whole U.S. population effectively. Thus, while we may lead the world in finding new treatments for AIDS, we lag in public health measures to halt the epidemic.

Opinion polls show that Americans realize that they are ill served by their health care system. While consumers and payers alike express dissatisfaction with health care, there is some ambivalence over the potential for reform to improve that care.[5] The depth of the dissatisfaction is hard to fathom, particularly for politicians and their advisers who have the 1992 and 1996 presidential elections in mind. One plausible scenario is that a continuing recession makes domestic issues the battleground for the presidential elections, and health care reform becomes politically irresistible. In this scenario, AIDS could be a catalyst for public calls for reform, perhaps by causing a collapse in a major urban hospital system.

AIDS could be just one of many developments pushing the political system toward health care reform, or it could become the trigger for political action. To date, the polity has responded only marginally to AIDS, but we are still early in the epidemic. When AIDS first struck the gay community, we had a conservative Republican administration elected with the help of the "moral majority." It was expedient to pay little attention to the disease. President Reagan did not talk about AIDS to the American public until 31 May 1987, after 20,849 Americans had died from the disease. He never mentioned gays in the speech.[6] The anger of the gay minority in this country was expressed in 1987 by Randy Shilts in his book *And the Bond Played On*:

> The numbers of AIDS cases measured the shame of the nation. . . . The United States, the one nation with the knowledge, the resources, and the institutions to respond to the epidemic, had failed. And it had failed because of ignorance and fear, prejudice and rejection. The story of the AIDS epidemic . . . was a story of bigotry and what it could do to a nation.[7]

In the 1990s, the growth in the number of AIDS cases will overcome a new population of victims—poor, minority users of illicit drugs and the people closest to them. These groups may be as marginal politically in the second phase of the epidemic as gays were in the first. As one public health expert notes:

> It has remained clear that the future course of the AIDS epidemic will be determined by the creation of a social and institutional milieu within which radical voluntary changes in behavior can occur and be sustained. Educational campaigns and counseling programs, most effectively undertaken by groups linked to the populations at risk, have remained the centerpiece of that preventive effort. . . . The most striking failure in the preventive realm, however, is rooted in the unwillingness to commit the resources necessary to treat drug abuse.[8]

While AIDS primarily hits politically marginal groups, most of the population, the media, and elected officials concentrate on other issues. It is easy to conclude, then, that AIDS will not trigger a movement for health care reform, at least until the epidemic threatens the general population in the political mainstream. This conclusion, however, ignores some of the challenges that AIDS will pose in a changing health care system.

NEW HEALTH CARE PARADIGM

AIDS will foment further change by exposing weaknesses in the most fundamental structure and practices of the health care system. The foundation of this system is a paradigm that was cracking even before the AIDS epidemic. Many of the twentieth-century health care concepts tied to this paradigm, which place sick people in hospitals and have doctors making medical decisions, are under attack. AIDS becomes one more force applying pressure to shift from the old paradigm described in Table 8–1 to a new paradigm. Unless the old paradigm creates a dramatic cure for AIDS or an effective vaccine in fairly short order, AIDS will likely be a strong force for a paradigm shift in health.

AIDS has unleashed a consumer movement that seeks the power, information, and choice that was assigned to higher authorities operating under the old paradigm. AIDS activists have created patient information networks, drug-purchasing groups, and a striking example of how motivated consumers can change health care. Regulatory authorities at the U.S. Food and Drug Administration were shocked by protesters who angrily rejected many fundamental rules of drug development. Physicians who treat AIDS and human immunodeficiency virus (HIV) infections have been surprised by patients who come to them knowing more about treatment options and experimental therapies than the doctors themselves. Pharmaceutical companies have been astounded that AIDS activists can gain access to corporate plans for developing drugs, using an underground of informants. The growing power of AIDS

TABLE 8–1   Characteristics of Old and New Health Care Paradigms

Old Paradigm	New Paradigm
Health is in the body	Health is spirit, mind, and body
Health equals absence of disease	Health equals maximum potentials and performance
Examines individuals	Examines society
Causal model	Multifactorial models
Pathogen focused	Systems view
Allopathic	Holistic
Physician dominated	Consumer oriented
Inpatient	Outpatient
Medical	Behavioral
Mass produced	Customized

groups had created more than just envy among other advocacy groups; it has created a model for activism.

If future AIDS activists from the inner cities take their cue from the current groups, then pressure will continue to push toward the new health care paradigm. In part, that shift is motivated by the desire to provide a more potent response to the rising epidemic. The new paradigm enlists all human resources in the struggle to thrive. The spirit and the mind are particularly important allies for HIV–infected individuals who may see victory not as eliminating the disease but as maintaining or recovering their self-esteem and their ability to function in spite of the disease. Some people with AIDS go so far as to place all their hope in faith healing or other approaches that are completely outside the traditional medical paradigm. Most people infected with HIV, however, do not ignore the offerings of the medical establishment; they just look for more than what medicine can offer.

BIOMEDICAL ADVANCES AND AIDS

Fortunately, biomedical advances will offer better treatment for AIDS. Molecular biology promises to achieve more in the next decades than in any previous era of scientific history. New tools—the scanning-tunneling microscope that can manipulate single atoms, supercomputers, monoclonal antibodies, and a raft of others—will help researchers create newer knowledge and discover new therapeutics. Molecular biology will enable scientists to model organ systems. The scientists will be able to create simulations so real that their experiments can mimic disease processes and then reveal therapeutic approaches.[9] The understanding of disease processes will open up enormous potential for designing new interventions.

Already AIDS provides a dramatic view of the speed and direction of basic research. So much has been learned about HIV in such a short time that

AIDS has itself become a force propelling research. Virologists can already describe the atomic structure of HIV, including the shape of the surface protein—gp 120—and the existence of two outer coats, called capsids. Their knowledge empowers other researchers to devise strategies to develop drugs that take advantage of the structure of HIV and, hopefully, to weaken or disarm it.[10] As more money pours into AIDS research, a scientific agenda that goes beyond AIDS comes into view. The frontiers of virology open not only to the study of retroviruses, but a host of other simple, relatively unknown life forms that will be implicated in a growing number of disease and life processes.

An even larger scientific agenda opens in immunology, where basic knowledge can be marshaled not just against AIDS but also against the larger, more established killers like cancers and heart disease. Immune system research continues advances in the allopathic approach, or reductionist research, which has achieved such impressive results as the characterization of key constituents in the immune system such as T-4 cells, macrophages, interleukins, and other cytokines. Undoubtedly, the positivistic and reductionist approach of traditional medical research will continue to add knowledge to the medical arsenal needed to fight AIDS.

This allopathic approach has, however, split the body and mind and focused on empirical research. Health care is thus set up to ignore what we can do with our minds, how our emotions affect our health and illness, and how our personal and spiritual growth can also affect our health. Scientific studies that use empirical research to explore these issues emerged rapidly in the 1990s from the field of psychoneuroimmunology. This research will encourage the use of what we describe as soft technologies, such as visualization and meditation.[11] Many people with AIDS will use soft technologies along with the latest drugs to both strengthen their immune response and attack the invading virus. These people will encourage a synthesis of the reductionist and holistic practices that are often in opposition to each other in current medical practice.

AIDS will also affect other areas where scientific progress is accelerating. Pharmacology has entered a new era that will be dominated by rational research rather than random searches for pharmacologically active compounds. With rational research, scientists begin with a knowledge of the disease process, human organ systems, and cells, right down to the molecular shape of receptors at the cellular level. With such knowledge, pharmacologists can look for molecules with the right shape to bind with receptors. They can manipulate atoms to create the right shape, eventually even designing drugs atom by atom.

This new research approach is expensive, however, and the new drugs that result will be far more expensive than older drugs. The first drug approved for AIDS, azidothymidine (AZT), shocked payers and patients alike with a price tag that most individuals simply cannot afford. AIDS groups have pressured manufacturers, politicians, and third-party payers to help make expensive drugs available. The issue of how to pay for increasingly expensive drugs will be more visible as new treatments for many different diseases are developed. AIDS could well be the disease, however, where activist patients have the capacity to confront the public with the need to change the financing system for drugs.

The new medicines developed later in this decade will be further enhanced by the understanding of genetics coming from the human genome project. The mapping of the human genome will affect every other type of biomedical research. Most powerfully, it will customize mass-produced knowledge about diseases to the biochemically unique characteristics of an individual person. Every drug on the market, whether for AIDS or any other condition, is developed for a statistical average patient. Doctors can adjust their prescribing to account for any individual variations that are known to affect how the drug works. To date, however, not much has been systematically learned about those individual variations. Some group factors such as race, age, and renal impairment are already known to affect drug response. Much more will be learned about group as well as individual difference when information from the genome project comes on line.[12]

The information systems that could take genetic knowledge into medical practice are revolutionary in themselves—AIDS can influence the course of the information revolution in health care because it raises crucial ethical and political issues. Even today's fragmented data bases, which are sure to look primitive in just a few years, frighten people with AIDS. The ownership of information about infected individuals is still open to question. Public health concerns clash with individual rights when AIDS registries are kept or when contact tracing notifies sexual partners of infected individuals. Insurance companies that test for HIV infection own the results, leaving the individual vulnerable to discrimination, loss of confidentiality, and laboratory error.

Given these current realities, the AIDS community must look carefully at new information systems capable of changing the delivery and financing of health care. On the positive side, the speed at which medical knowledge accumulates and improves medical practice could increase dramatically with new information systems. The computer-based patient record, for example, is "an essential technology for health care" for which there are no technological developmental barriers.[13] Health outcome measures are also developing that could link health care inputs with multidimensional outcomes, including cost, health status, and quality-of-life dimensions. In addition, expert systems for diagnosis and treatment protocols show great promise for establishing standards of care.

Taken together, these technologies have the potential to empower patients. The complexity of medicine will no longer make the notion of the informed consumer of health care an unrealizable ideal. The coming generations of computers will cope with the complexity for people. Patients conceivably will be able to use computers instead of physicians as the "learned intermediaries" who guide health decisions. There will still be important roles for physicians and other professionals as healers, health coaches, and perhaps guides for decision making, but the roles will change and so too will the rules of the system. If consumers use the emerging information systems to gain decision-making power, physicians will lose the monopoly that is granted them through licensure. Yet, doctors are also likely to lose their terrible liability burden as well. Patients will have to accept the risks and responsibilities that are unavoidably a part of the ongoing experiment we call medicine.

If medicine is an experiment, it has been limited by the fact that most results are not systematically collected to create new knowledge. The health care system of the twenty-first century will have a capacity to gather an enormous amount of data to answer questions we cannot even ask now. Twenty-four-hour monitoring; lifelong data bases on behavior, environment, genetics, and health care; and artificial-intelligence tools called knowbots and knowledge navigators that search all medical knowledge to answer an individual's question are some of the bright possibilities now seen by the visionaries in medicine.

There is, however, a darker side to the technological potential of information systems. The specter of information systems used against individuals rather than disease evokes images from Orwell and Kafka. Individuals with the AIDS virus could, conceivably, not know they are infected; they could suffer from discrimination based upon health records they never see. With advancing genetic information available through tests, this type of discrimination could broaden beyond AIDS to affect people having predispositions to any number of diseases. Even the threat of such abuses of medical confidentiality could be used by established interests to block their loss of power to the emerging information infrastructure.

These essentially political issues contribute to the great uncertainty facing our health care system as it responds to the AIDS epidemic. As futurists, our response to uncertainty is to explore the range of potential changes using alternative scenarios. These scenarios help point to the key choices facing our society, including those defining the delivery, financing, and use of technology.

The way that our society makes these choices by formulating policy is itself changing. Policy makes things happen. Tools are emerging that allow us to explore what might happen far more effectively. These include the type of futures research that the Institute for Alternative Futures and other health futurists provide.

But equally important, since we continually create the future by what we do and what we fail to do, is the emergence of processes for the development of our vision. Vision in this context is what we see with our eyes closed, that is, our preferred future, the future we want to create. Work on visions in a number of public and private sector organizations has shown that a great deal of personal power can be unleashed if people share a vision of the positive role their organization is playing and if attention is being given to using visioning techniques to enhance the conscious, inspiring, and compelling creation of a society that reflects our deepest values.

What should our vision be? This question becomes an invitation to design the best that can be. In health care, our vision is to move away from an expensive, often insensitive, narrowly focused health care system. We see the possibility of a system that is more caring and more focused on prevention; a system that helps each individual manage health, healing with the body and the mind; a system that measures what works in order to keep learning more about health; a system that recognizes the inevitability of death and helps us prepare for it. AIDS is one of the challenges that will help create such a health care system.

NOTES

1. Throughout this article, we will use the term "AIDS" to encompass not only diagnosed disease but also infection with the human immunodeficiency virus and disease related to this virus.

2. George J. Schieber, Jean-Pierre Poullier, and Leslie M. Greenwald, "Health Care Systems in Twenty-Four Countries," *Health Affairs*, 10(3):24 (Fall 1991).

3. Jeffrey Goldsmith, Ph.D., coined this description of the approach of modern medicine to disease.

4. Schieber, Poullier, and Greenwald, "Health Care Systems," pp. 34–37.

5. Cindy Jajich-Toth and Burns W. Roper, "Americans' Views on Health Care: A Study in Contradictions," *Health Affairs*, 9(4):149–57 (Winter 1990). See also Joel C. Cantor et al., "Business Leaders' Views on American Health Care," *Health Affairs*, 10(1):98–105 (Spring 1991).

6. Randy Shilts, *And the Band Played On* (New York: St. Martin's Press, 1987), p. 596.

7. Ibid., p. 601.

8. Ronald Bayer, "AIDS: The Politics of Prevention and Neglect," *Health Affairs*, 10(1):93 (Spring 1991).

9. Peck and Rabin, *Regulating Change*, p. 19.

10. See, for example, Ron Cowen, "The Shell Game: A Common Cold Virus Offers Clues to Sabotaging AIDS," *Science News*, 28 July 1990, pp. 56–57.

11. Clement Bezold, Rick J. Carlson, and Jonathan C. Peck, *The Future of Work and Health* (Dover, MA: Auburn House, 1986), pp. 125–31.

12. Peck and Rabin, *Regulating Change*, p. 25.

13. Institute of Medicine, *The Computer-Based Patient Record: An Essential Technology for Health Care* (Washington, DC: National Academy Press, 1991).

PART THREE

The International-Comparative Dimension of AIDS

9

Responding to AIDS: Governmental Policy Responses

Stella Z. Theodoulou

During the last few years the study of the politics and policy of acquired immune deficiency syndrome (AIDS) has become more prevalent; however, a body of literature that deals with the comparative analysis of governmental policies on AIDS is absent. What do exist are limited or individual country case studies (Ballard, 1992; Berridge & Strong, 1990; Day & Klein, 1989; Freeman, 1992; Kirp & Bayer, 1992; Misztal & Moss, 1990; Moerkerk & Aggleton, 1990; Pollak, 1993). The argument in favor of comparative study is strong and, as Weeks (1990, p.13) argues, AIDS provides a golden opportunity to look at the complexities of policy formation in pluralist societies.

From the existing literature common features may be discerned in how different governments have responded to the AIDS epidemic. First, in no country in the first years of the epidemic was there a coherent national policy. This was due in large part to the scientific uncertainties surrounding the virus. Second, in most nations, nongovernmental organizations were formed in the communities that were most concerned/affected by AIDS. Only after this had occurred and there was political recognition of the epidemic's severity did governments enter the policy arena on AIDS (Pollock et al., 1993; Mann et al., 1992). Next, AIDS first appeared in an economic down period and thus increasing responsibility was placed on the private sector rather than public sector in human immunodeficiency virus (HIV)/AIDS policy research and treatment. Fourth, before actual government mobilization, most nations had in place preexisting public health mechanisms dealing with sexually transmitted diseases. Fifth, the first policy centered mainly on programs that dealt with screening and testing issues. Sixth, after 1988 the problem for AIDS activists in most nations was how to maintain the salience of the AIDS issue on the policy agenda. Seventh, with the onset of government funding, there was a process of routinization and normalization around the AIDS issue that led to the virus being perceived as a chronic rather than an epidemic disease. Eighth, policy responses in each nation have been shaped by the existing policy tradition in the social and health policy areas. Ninth, most national strategies to deal with AIDS have been formulated as cautions (Misztal & Moss 1990, pp. 234–49). Finally, in most countries governmental inaction has been justified by the association of AIDS with marginalized and stigmatized groups within the society.

POLICY SCHEMES

Most authors agree with Kirp and Bayer (1992) that despite their similarities in AIDS policy not all countries have responded in the same manner. Although Kirp and Bayer's analysis is confined to Western industrialized nations, their conclusions also can be applied to many developing nations of the world. From the analysis of eleven industrialized nations, Kirp and Bayer argue that public policy on AIDS is unique to each nation, its politics, and culture. Thus, if we want to understand a nation's AIDS policy we must try to first look at the characteristics of that nation's culture and how it deals with matters of sexuality, sexual relations, drug use, privacy, minority rights, and perceived threats to public health. If such an approach is taken when looking at a number of nations then it is possible to see that this has been a diversity of policy responses to the AIDS problem. For example, in the United States, the United Kingdom, Sweden, and Australia, governmental AIDS information campaigns stress the fear of death, whereas in the Netherlands, France, Spain, and Denmark the mortality aspect is almost completely ignored (Misztal & Moss, 1990). In the United States and Australia gay bathhouses were either closed or regulated, whereas they were allowed to stay open with certain restrictions in the Netherlands and Denmark. Needle exchange programs are accepted without argument in the Netherlands but have aroused bitter controversy and division in Germany and the United States.

Although AIDS policy decisions cannot be reduced to a single simple formulation, Kirp and Bayer suggest that most nation's responses fall somewhere between two strategies (Kirp & Bayer, 1992). The first is the contain-and-control approach that emphasizes compulsory identification and isolation of HIV–infected individuals. Such an approach is based on late nineteenth century public health practices and is the basis of many European nations' responses to sexually transmitted diseases in the post 1914 period. The second strategy is the cooperation-and-inclusion approach. This stresses cooperation, through education, voluntary testing, and counseling programs, with those individuals who are most susceptible to AIDS, while protecting their civil rights and privacy. Although this is part of a newer trend in public health policy, it has been used in the post–1960 era to fight chronic noninfectious diseases that are linked to behavioral patterns (alcoholism, lung disease, and heart disease). The emphasis is on the modification of behavior and thus lifestyle.

In most nations there has been a debate about which strategy and approach to AIDS policymaking should be adopted. Overall, the policy responses of most nations are somewhere between the two, although elements of each approach are present in varying degrees in all nations' policies. For the most part policy decisions reflect the balance of political forces in the nation and the dominant values and commitment of society to privacy and liberty. As Kirp and Bayer (1992, p. 5) conclude, "the politics of AIDS is the politics of Democracy in the face of a critical challenge to communal well being."

Michael Pollak, although using different labels, comes to similar conclusions. He also argues that there are two policy strategies a country can adopt. Governments have the option to choose to formulate liberal vs. coercive policies (Pollak, 1993, p. 56). Liberal policies are based on respect for anonymity and voluntariness rather than coercion. Coercive policies require compulsory regulation of behavior and carry penalties for violation of rules. Which policy a nation selects depends on the level of consensus politics present in its polity. For example, in the United Kingdom political consensus has organized around a liberal AIDS policy conception. Thus, AIDS has been largely omitted from traditional party conflict. Most of Europe has followed suit (Pollak, 1993, p. 56–59). This is different from the United States, where Quam and Ford (1990, p. 33–36) conclude many states have extended to public health authorities the ability to confine, isolate, and quarantine people with AIDS, and where the virus has been added to traditional sexually transmitted disease (STD) legislation and to antisodomy legislation that exists in about fifty percent of the states. The difference between the liberal and coercive approaches is best seen in the way in which the United States and the European community legislate travel and immigration for HIV/AIDS individuals. In the United States AIDS was added to the list of contagious diseases that precludes access to America (Quam and Ford, 1990, p. 31). The European community has denounced such regulation as discrimination and undemocratic.

Pollak's coercive scheme bears obvious similarities to Kirp and Bayer's contain-and-control policymaking, while his liberal policy definition clearly correlates to Kirp and Bayer's cooperation-and-inclusion type. Whichever label one wishes to choose, we can conclude that all nations obviously face a dilemma when attempting to deal with the demands of the AIDS epidemic. The dilemma is how can the spread of infection be controlled while civil and human rights are protected. Research seems to demonstrate that industrial nations have tried to find a balance. In certain nations discriminatory practices and violations of rights have occurred; however, no industrialized democracy has chosen a solely repressive policy to handle the epidemic. In other words, although many countries have elements of coercion in their policies, no industrialized nation has chosen mandatory testing and quarantine of people with AIDS. This is a clear rejection of the coercive strategy. Analysis of developing nations presents a somewhat different picture (Hendriks & Knichler, 1991; Leiner, 1994).

CONCLUSION

When looking at industrialized nations' responses to AIDS we can conclude that cultural and political norms have helped to shape governmental responses to the epidemic. National values affect how a nation defines and understands AIDS, and this, in turn, impacts on a government's ability to take certain actions. Randy Shilts (1987), argues the homosexual link to AIDS was overlooked by European scientists because they were not as culturally obsessed with alternative lifestyles as their American counterparts, and this is reflected in the way the epidemic has been handled on a policymaking level.

AIDS policymaking has not been static, and thus responses have not remained the same. However, all nations' responses follow similar patterns or stages. In the early years AIDS was an open policy arena with no established policy mechanisms or recognized "policy community" around the disease. Policy input was from below with the formation of a new policy community consisting of groups outside the normal policymaking process. This new community was composed of gay activists, clinicians, scientists, and those who had lost loved ones to the epidemic. What united this community was the shared belief of the need for urgent government action and the dangers of a "lurking" menace of heterosexual transmission. This stage eventually gave way in the late eighties to the national emergencies period. In this stage AIDS became a priority and no government could afford to be perceived as sitting back and doing nothing. The nineties has seen a third stage of routinization and normalization. Thus AIDS with the advent of government funding and policy has become part and parcel of most nations' public health sectors domain. With this development AIDS is no longer viewed as an epidemic, but rather as a chronic disease that society must live with. Thus, policies for the most part have not been coercive, but have relied on education and volunteerism. In the upcoming years the priority of AIDS activists must be to keep the issue high on the policy agenda. What must be undertaken now is a comparative analysis of less-developed regions of the world and their policy responses.

REFERENCES

Ballard, J. (1992). Australia, participation and innovation in a federal system, in Kirp, D. L., & Bayer, R., eds. *AIDS in the Industrialized Democracies.* New Brunswick: Rutgers University Press.

Berridge, V. (1991). AIDS, the media and health policy. *Heath Education Journal*, 50.4: pp. 179–85.

Berridge, V., & Strong, P. (1990). AIDS policies in the U.K., in Fee, E., & Fox, D., eds. *AIDS: Contemporary History*. Princeton, N.J.: Princeton University Press.

Day, P., & Klein, R. (1989). Interpreting the unexpected: the case of AIDS policy making in Britain. *Journal of Public Policy*, 9.3: pp. 337–53.

Freeman, R. (1992). The politics of AIDS in Britain and Germany, in Aggleton, P., Davies, P., & Hart, G. *AIDS: Rights, Risk and Reason*. London: Falmer Press.

Hendriks, A., & Knichler, K. (May 1991). About turn in Central and Eastern Europe, *World AIDS*, pp. 7–15.

Kirp, D.L., & Bayer, R. (1992). *AIDS in the Industrialized Democracies*. New Brunswick: Rutgers University Press.

Leiner, M. (1994). *Sexual Politics in Cuba: Machismo, Homosexuality and AIDS*. Boulder: Westview Press.

Mann, J.M., Tarantola, D.J.M., & Netler, T.W., eds. (1992). *AIDS in the Third World*. Cambridge, MA: Harvard University Press.

Misztal, B.A., & Moss, D., eds. (1990). *Action on AIDS: National Policies in Comparative Perspective*. New York: Greenwood.

Moerkerk, H., & Aggleton, P. (1990). AIDS prevention strategies in Europe: a comparison and critical analysis, in Aggleton, P., Davies, P., & Hart, G. *AIDS: Individual Cultural and Policy Dimensions*. Lewes: Falmer Press.

Pollak, M. (1992). AIDS in West Germany: coordinating policy in a federal system, in Kirp, D.L., & Bayer R., eds. *AIDS in the Industrialized Democracies*. New Brunswick: Rutgers University Press.

Pollak, M. (1993). *The Second Plague of Europe: AIDS Prevention and Sexual Transmission Among Men in Western Europe*. Binghamton, N.Y.: Harrington Park.

Pollock, P., Lillie, S., & Vittes, M. (March 1993). On the nature and dynamics of social construction: the case of AIDS. *Social Science Quarterly*, pp. 123–35.

Quam, M., & Ford, N. (1990). AIDS policies and practices in the United States, in Mitzal, B., & Moss, D., eds. *Action on AIDS: National Policies in Comparative Perspective*. New York: Greenwood Press.

Shilts, R. (1987). *And the Band Played on: Politics, People, and the AIDS Epidemic*. New York: Penguin Books.

Weeks, J. (1990). AIDS: the intellectual agenda, in Aggleton, P., Davies, P., & Hart, G. *AIDS: Individual Cultural and Policy Dimensions*. Lewes: Falmer Press.

10

AIDS: Cuba's Effort to Contain

Marvin Leiner

We have the opportunity to stop the disease in our country. It would be irresponsible if we didn't face the situation with courage, knowing we could stop it. We have an epidemiologic opportunity that we are not going to lose.
—Dr. Hector Terry

In Cuba, AIDS has not become a dilemma, a social problem, a phobia, a madness, as in the United States.
—Reynaldo González

In Cuba, the medical establishment's response to AIDS was immediate and thorough; its goal was to prevent an epidemic by identifying, isolating, and treating, to the extent medically possible, all persons infected with the HIV virus, whether or not they had developed AIDS. To this end, mandatory screening for HIV infection began in 1986, and persons testing positive were sent to a sanitorium in a Havana suburb. The first blood tests targeted the most high-risk groups: Cubans who had traveled abroad in various capacities since 1975; in particular, soldiers who had served in Africa.

By April 1991, 9,771,691 people, almost the entire population, had been tested. Almost two years later, a cumulative total of 13 million tests had been carried out as people in high-risk groups began to undergo repeated tests.[1]

Twelve special sanitoriums are now in operation throughout the country. As of December 1, 1992, 862 positive HIV cases had been detected. Three months later the number was up to 902. One hundred fifty nine have developed AIDS, and, of these, 119 have died including two children.[2]

To achieve this medical success, the primary aim has been to identify infected persons and bring them completely under the control of the medical establishment. Education has been relegated to a marginal role. Although people living in a sanitorium receive (at no cost to them) the best possible medical treatment and have comfortable living conditions, their quarantine is obligatory. They must live isolated, nonproductive lives until they contract AIDS and are moved to a hospital, or until a miracle cure is found. Already some people have lived almost seven years in this state of limbo. It amounts to a life sentence for healthy people. Although it is difficult to know how long it will take for a person to progress from HIV infection to symptoms of AIDS, studies have shown that the median time is ten and one-half years. Some people testing HIV–positive may not develop AIDS for twenty years. Indeed, with excellent medical care and early intervention with present drugs and more powerful ones yet to be developed, researchers state that the hope is "that it will take longer and longer before symptoms occur and that some people may never become ill at all."[3] And, even with improved testing procedures, there is still some chance of false positives.

THE QUARANTINE POLICY

> The sanitorium is also the most viable solution for a poor country like Cuba, so that resources can be focused efficiently in efforts to keep the disease from spreading indiscriminately. The way we see it, we must also protect the human rights of the majority of the population.
>
> —Dr. Hector Terry

> All of these reasons lead us to believe that the prevalence of the HIV among the Cuban population is really very low and that it is mainly due to the nationwide program which allows for relatively early detection and to isolation of those detected to keep it from spreading in geometric proportions.
>
> —Editorial, *Weekly Granma*

The most controversial aspect of Cuba's program for combatting AIDS has been the creation of sanitoriums for the compulsory isolation of those Cubans who test positive for HIV antibodies. While there have been discussions in other countries about instituting such a national quarantine for those identified as infected, Cuba's is the only one of its kind in the world. People admitted to a sanitorium have the virus but do not have AIDS. People with AIDS are hospitalized.

The first sanitorium opened in Havana in April 1986 with 24 patients. It is now the largest of the twelve sanitoriums with 300 patients; another five regional sanitoriums are under construction.[4] The first director of the sanitorium, Dr. Juan Rivero Gómez, currently heads the medical department, which is made up of three wards—observation, psychiatry, and dental. In addition, there are four clinics. Every Friday, specialists see patients for whatever problems they may have.

The Sanitorium

The Havana sanitorium is located near the city of Santiago de las Vegas, a residential resort area known as Los Cocos. Visitors to the facility of forty hectares have described the residents' living quarters as apartments, which include color television, air conditioning, and kitchen facilities.[5] The most attractive part of the sanitorium is El Maranon, an area with two-story houses near the main entrance. El Maranon is the community for the most "responsible" patients—married couples or two patients of the same sex living together. Patients receive the weekly food ration, which they prepare as they wish.[6]

Upon first arrival, patients are interviewed by physicians and nurse specialists—epidemiologists. There is, according to public health officials, an emphasis on both the "personal" and the "communal."

> Once a person is diagnosed, an interview takes place at which his/her situation is set forth. "You have the AIDS virus," the person is told. It is as if a twenty-story building had fallen upon the person. The person is informed that there is no effective treatment.
>
> It is explained that there are enormous financial, human, and technological resources throughout the world dedicated to the study of the disease—dedicated to the pursuit of a vaccine that will prevent the disease, to seeking a drug or an effective pharmacological agent to treat this disease, but that at the present time none of this is available.
>
> . . .The person is told that there is no way to protect the life of those who carry the virus at present other than to protect them from the aggressions of the environment. . . . It is a somewhat individualistic focus . . . directed to make the person understand that this measure is taken for his/her own good. It is like putting him/her in internment for a while until the solution to the problem appears, whether it be one year, two years, or longer.
>
> And the other aspect is the social aspect. If you are infected, you may infect others.[7]

The interview data gathered for each person include family history, housing, work history, and present work situation, including salary. Patients continue to receive full salary even though not working. Arrangements are made to enable university students to continue their studies.

In the sanitorium, married couples and homosexual couples live together if both have tested positive. Uninfected children then live with other family members rather than with their parents. If the children are also infected, they join their parents in the sanitorium. If only one parent tests positive, that parent lives in the sanitorium, and children continue living with the other parent; family members and friends can visit those living in the sanitorium any time they choose.

On staff, working closely with residents, are health professionals trained to work with HIV–positive people. In order to provide continuity of treatment and a personal connection to the resident, a physician is assigned to each patient (the term health officials use to denote a resident of the sanitorium). A team of psychologists, social workers, and sociologists not only work with the patients but meet with and provide counseling and psychiatric services for family members. Families are encouraged to visit as often as every day.

Residents of the sanitorium may also make trips outside. There are occasional organized recreational activities such as an evening at the cinema or the theater or an outing to the beach. Residents also return to their communities for visits and meetings—for example, of the block association or parent-teacher conferences. Those who do not live far away can spend weekends with family and friends. If they do live farther away, they can arrange four-day trips home every four to six weeks.

On most of these trips, a senior medical student or intern goes along as chaperone because, as the director of the Havana sanitorium explained, "Our responsibility doesn't end at the doors of the institution; we must see to the health of everyone."[8] Dr. Terry says,"Our objective is not to have them lead an isolated existence, but to find a way to keep them from developing the disease and from spreading it to other parts of the population."[9] He has also explained that "those hospitalized in the sanitorium continue to have sexual relations with their partners if they so desire"[10] when they go home on weekends. Presumably, these partners are considered as good as infected, since the whole point of the sanitorium and chaperoned visits is to prevent sexual contacts that could spread the virus. Married couples are allowed passes to leave the sanitorium under more liberal conditions than others and are not required to be chaperoned.[11]

The new director at the Havana facility, Dr. Jorge Pérez Avila, seeks to identify stable and responsible couples and individuals who can be trusted to return to normal life in the community without engaging in behavior that will put others at risk. Pérez reported to the "First Seminar on HIV Infection and AIDS in Cuba" (*Primer Seminario Sobre Infección Por VIH y SIDA en Cuba*) held in Havana on October 30–31, 1992 that the quarantine program is now more flexible.[12]

Thus far, a handful of people have been deemed responsible enough to return to society, and about half those residing in the Havana sanitorium may now leave on unchaperoned weekend visits. Being among these requires approval by a group of psychologists, medical personnel, and social workers who consider epidemiological records, psychiatric data, relations with family members, and the person's behavior while at the sanitorium. A person is not eligible for this "parole" until he or she has lived in the sanitorium for at least six months. Thus, the quarantine is eased for people who are HIV positive and are "responsible." But, what is "responsible" or "trustworthy?" This is an Orwellian/Catch-22 nightmare. If you're a homosexual resident in a sanitorium and put on makeup or are considered "effeminate," is this "irresponsible?" If you protest sanitorium conditions, does that mean that you will be designated "untrustworthy?" If you protest or object to the entire quarantine concept for HIV positives, is this also "untrustworthy" and "irresponsible?"

Dr. Fernando Zakarias of the Pan American Health Organization's AIDS division has visited the sanitoriums regularly. He reports that the Cubans "have psychologists who do tests and claim to be able to prove at the outset who is trustworthy. We say 'How can you do this? Unless someone is a clear sociopath, how can you tell?' " He further states that the Cubans find most homosexual residents of the sanitoriums "untrustworthy."[13]

Indeed, the process is much like that of release from a mental hospital. No doubt a few people testing HIV-positive are mentally ill, and no doubt a few are highly promiscuous with no sense of concern for their sexual partners. The process, however, seems to assume that to test HIV–positive is to be mentally unstable and irresponsible until proven otherwise through a rigorous process.

Carlos Cabrera, who reported on the sanitorium for the *Weekly Granma*, thought it would not be easy for these people to return to society because of prejudice and the lack of education about AIDS. "Reintegration into the society is also difficult because Cubans have reacted with panic to AIDS."[14]

Thus, when sanitorium residents go out on visits, people they encounter often feel endangered. One woman resident described to a North American journalist in Havana an encounter she had with an old friend who would not believe she was a sanitorium patient. "I couldn't convince her I was serious." She went on to describe an evening at the Tropicana night club:

> There were two young men at the next table. One of them was telling the other, "You know, you have to be really careful on Sundays, because that's when they let the 'siderosos'[15] out." I turned around quickly and must have glared at him, because he said somewhat defensively, "Excuse me, Ma'am, but it's true. You should be careful too." I don't have to be careful, I told him, because I already have AIDS. The young man said: "Señora, you shouldn't joke about things like that."[16]

The Testing Program

Given the growing international epidemic the Cuban Ministry of Health ordered a screening process that would eventually test virtually every person on the island for the infection. It began in 1986 when all blood donors were tested. At that time, 17 carriers of the virus, or .0026 percent, were found, according to Deputy Health Minister Hector Terry.[17] Among Cubans having contact with foreigners, one of the first major groups tested were troops, aid workers, and technicians returning from Angola. By 1989, this included 300,000 Cubans, among whom 82, or .0002 percent, tested HIV–positive. In addition, all Cubans returning from abroad were tested, whether they were diplomats, athletes, sailors, soldiers, or students.

Testing also began on citizens having contact with foreigners in Cuba, whether in education, tourism, or foreign relations. Hotel and restaurant workers in the tourist industry, for example, are considered a high-risk group. All foreigners who reside in Cuba for three months or longer are now tested, except for diplomats. Tourists are not tested. Anyone who tests positive is returned to his or her country of origin.[18]

Early on, the mandatory testing program expanded to include all pregnant women, all adults admitted to hospitals, people treated for sexually transmitted diseases, the sexual contacts of those testing HIV–positive, and prisoners. There has also been some screening of specific residential areas where an initial high proportion of HIV–infected people were found or where there was a high level of tourist activity. Ultimately, all members of the armed forces will be tested.

In the absence of a serious educational program on AIDS, the quarantine itself becomes a kind of collective safe sex program that requires that infected people remove themselves from society so society can remain untainted. This also explains why people rarely refuse to cooperate with the quarantine and what happens when they do. Most people accept the need to protect society, and since the quarantine policy was put into place early on by high-level authorities, it preempted consideration of other possibilities. People cannot imagine either an alternative or any way to achieve one. Some GNTES staff have indicated that, although they did not agree with the quarantine, they did not feel they could actively oppose it. And, after a while, who argues with success? Nationwide testing and quarantine have kept AIDS at a very low level.

To gain compliance from those testing positive becomes a matter of paternalistic persuasion rather than force—as is obvious in several health ministry statements in response to questions of noncompliance. In a 1988 interview, health care officials stated that there were no refusals because when one learns one is infected, one is in a fog and can be convinced to accept the painful logic of isolating oneself for the good of family and nation.[19]

Diego Franchi, a psychologist at the Havana sanitorium, explained to Carlos Cabrera of *Granma* that patients at the sanitorium go through three stages: first, denying one is sick; second, refusing to acknowledge it publicly; third, accepting one's condition and cooperating with medical staff.[20] Since most of the people he is talking about are not sick, denial is understandable even as they come to understand what it means to test positive for HIV. It is also understandable they would not want it publicly known given public attitudes about "diseased people who are such a social menace they must be put away." Finally, the third stage seems like one of defeat: there is no other place to turn. This feeling was expressed by Dr. Terry in response to a question on whether people tried to escape from the sanitorium.

> Some patients have left the sanitorium. It's easy to do since this is a health facility, not a prison, and so therefore has only the most elementary physical measures for containment that any other health facility should have. The patients who left have gone to their homes; they did not try to evade health authorities so the term "capture" is inappropriate. All we did is locate them at their homes and convince them that in doing so, they are only harming their own health.
>
> There are some people who at first refused to go to the sanitorium. We simply kept talking to them until they were convinced of the necessity of in-patient care. There are, however, health regulations in our country that would allow health officials to take measures against anyone who was endangering the health of the general population in their community.[21]

IMPEDIMENTS TO ALTERNATIVE POLICIES

Why has Cuba—outstanding for its achievements in education and for its emphasis on education as the solution to many problems of underdevelopment—been almost the only country not to make education the central or dominant element in its anti–AIDS strategy? The reason lies, I think, in a convergence of five conditions:

1. The nation's successful development of a highly technical and advanced health care system providing free services to all citizens;
2. The fear generated by an epidemic that appears to be uncontrollable and feeds on public ignorance;
3. The pervasiveness of machismo and its general rejection of sex education;
4. An authoritarian political system in which voices that might advocate alternative policies are not allowed the means to organize and present their case;
5. The strong prejudice against homosexuality and the perception of AIDS as a homosexual disease.

Cuba's Advanced Health Care System

Cuba's health care system has, as I have discussed, won respect in international health communities. Death and infant mortality rates are among the lowest in the world; indeed, infant mortality is the lowest among all Third World countries. Several diseases common to nonindustrial countries have been eliminated. Medical care is available even in the remotest regions of the country. Cuba's community doctor program, a doctor for every 120 families, has earned the interest and admiration of doctors and health workers throughout the world.[22] This small island nation has become a medical power admired by most Third World countries for the availability of free medical care and the development of medical technology on a par with industrialized countries.

Some American physicians and health experts have criticized "Cuba's excessive use of doctors and the government's reliance on highly trained physicians to perform tasks that can be done by paraprofessionals." They fear an overemphasis on physician care that dangerously inflates the cost of health care. "Nevertheless, the Cuban health care system has accomplished what few if any of the other 100 developing nations of the world—and many industrialized countries—have attained."[23]

These advances made it possible to offer AIDS patients and those testing HIV–positive the best in medical care. The first steps in Cuba's anti–AIDS strategy were taken in 1983 when blood and blood products from countries with AIDS cases were not permitted to enter the country. The Cubans, aware that blood concentrates needed in the treatment of hemophiliac bleeding are a major source of HIV infection in Latin America, stopped importing them from the East or the West. After a visit to Cuba in the early 1980s, Jeanne Smith and Sergio Piomelli, hematologists and professors of medicine and pediatrics at Columbia University's College of Physicians and Surgeons, reported that the Cubans

> started on their own to manufacture cryoprecipitate, a less purified blood fraction used several years ago, less efficient than the concentrates, but much less likely to be contaminated with HIV. This was no minor effort for a small country; during the night trucks still ferry the plasma from blood banks throughout the island to a central laboratory. Today, only four out of 500 hemophiliacs in Cuba are HIV carriers. By contrast, in the United States, the vast majority of hemophiliacs became HIV carriers in the early 1980s, and hundreds have died of AIDS.[24]

Ironically, the United States policy of prohibiting shipment of medical supplies and products, including blood, to Cuba unintentionally protected Cuban hemophiliacs. Officials state that Cuba is now almost completely self-sufficient in its blood supply.[25]

Because all health care for all citizens in Cuba is free, the cost of treating seriously ill people, including those with AIDS, does not become a hellish economic crisis that depletes income, is next to impossible to manage, and degrades patient, family, and friends in the process. In Cuba all hospital stays, doctor's treatment, and medication are free. For example, those who become ill with AIDS are treated in hospitals and receive medications such as AZT (at a cost of $7,000 per patient per year) at no cost to themselves. A number of asymptomatic patients at the sanitorium have been treated with Interferon; the results are encouraging but not conclusive. As Paula Treichler notes in her work on AIDS and HIV infection in the Third World: "One can certainly argue that Cuba is providing more support and resources for its infected citizens than many other countries."[26]

In Puerto Rico, on the other hand, federal records for the year ending March 31, 1990, show that it had the highest incidence of new AIDS cases of any place under U.S. government jurisdiction—47 new cases per 100,000 people.

Yet the few facilities offering care do not offer AZT to patients because it is too expensive. Dr. Samuel A. Amill explained that at the nineteen-bed adult ward of the AIDS Institute, no one received AZT "because if we give it to one, we should give it to everybody, and that would consume the Institute's whole budget."[27]

The centralized structure of Cuba's health care system makes it feasible to carry out an ongoing massive national testing program. This, in itself, generates a propensity to approach the disease only in medical technological terms. Reliance on a medical approach alone is no doubt influenced also by knowledge that AIDS is a rapidly spreading worldwide epidemic. Thus, strong measures must be taken as rapidly as possible lest the disease become uncontrollable.

The Cuban AIDS Screening Program

In Cuba, the testing program and necessary census procedures were carried out with the support of the mass organizations. The same organizations that had been the key to mobilization for the literacy and education campaigns and for the giant vaccination and health campaigns again helped with the screening program for AIDS.

In addition to government agencies, the Cuban Trade Unions (CTC), the Federation of Cuban Women (FMC), and the block organizations—the Committees for the Defense of the Revolution—all helped gather information for the census: for example, compiling lists of persons who had been outside of Cuba since 1975.

By October 1988, after almost two and a half years, nearly three million Cubans had been tested for the HIV virus—approximately 30 percent of the nation's population. During the following two and a half years, the rate of testing more than doubled so that an additional 6,839,442 were tested.[28] Those in high-risk groups are tested more than once.

At a 1989 meeting on AIDS in Latin America sponsored by the Pan American Health Organization, experts acknowledged that Cuba's screening was proportionally the largest in the world. The Cuban AIDS infection rate is one of the lowest in the world and the lowest in Latin America.[29]

Table 5-1 presents the infection rate within the specific groups tested for HIV as of 1989. Thus, the largest percentage of persons infected, 4.6 percent, was from the group of "sexual contacts of seropositive persons." Sexual contacts of HIV-positive Cubans are retested every three months and offered counseling services.[30] When questioned about intravenous drug users, officials said there were none in Cuba. I have been unable to find evidence to contradict these statements.

The smallest percentage of people with the HIV virus came from the category of pregnant women—.0037 percent. All women receive free prenatal care. If routine blood tests reveal the HIV virus, a woman may choose to have an abortion. As of 1990, only one child had died of AIDS. I have received one unconfirmed report that two HIV positive women chose to take the risk of giv-

TABLE 5–1 1989 Infection Rate Within Specific Groups Tested for HIV in Cuban Population

Groups Tested	Percentage of Infection Within Designated Group
Foreign students	.44
Persons with hemophilia	.3
Those who have lived outside Cuba since 1975	.025
Patients with sexually transmitted diseases	.010
The general population of resort areas	.005
Pregnant women	.0037
Sexual contacts of seropositive persons	4.6
A residual category (including prisoners)	.014
1989 total seroprevalence since testing began in 1986 (N=259)	.0089

Source: Francisco A. Machado Ramírez, director of the Cuban AIDS Investigations Laboratory, cited in Ronald Bayer and Cheryl Healton, "Special Report: Controlling AIDS in Cuba," *The New England Journal of Medicine,* April 13, 1989. p. 1023.

ing birth.[31] If so, they are in a no-win dilemma. The mothers must take up life in one of the sanitoriums; if the babies do not carry the virus, they must be brought up by someone else, although there can be frequent visits between mother and child. Only if the child is also infected can it join its mother in the sanitorium.

Table 5–2 presents the incidence of AIDS in Caribbean countries with populations of more than 100,000. Table 5–3 presents the incidence of AIDS

TABLE 5–2 Cumulative Incidence of AIDS in Caribbean Countries with Populations of More Than 100,000, October 1990

Country	Rate per Million
Bahamas	2,006
Guadaloupe	650
Trinidad and Tobago	540
Barbados	494
Martinique	409
Haiti	397
St. Vincent and the Grenadines	203
Dominican Republic	198
Grenada	170
Saint Lucia	120
Jamaica	66
Cuba	6.2

Source: Jens J. Pindborg, Department of Oral Pathology, Royal Dental College, Copenhagen, Denmark, "Global Aspects of the AIDS Epidemic," *Oral Surgery, Oral Medicine, Oral Pathology,* 73(1992): 139. Data in the table is based on the *WHO Weekly Epidemiological Record,* No. 40, October 5, 1990. Reprinted by permission.

TABLE 5–3 Cumulative Incidence of AIDS in
Selected Countries, October 1990

Country	Rate per Million
Congo	1,021
Uganda	724
United States	589
Zaire	379
France	174
Canada	170
Spain	159
Australia	118
Brazil	77
U.K.	60
Mexico	53
Venezuela	46
Argentina	23
Cuba	6.2

Source: Adapted from Jens J. Pindborg, Department of
Oral Pathology, Royal Dental College, Copenhagen,
Denmark, "Global Aspects of the AIDS Epidemic," *Oral
Surgery, Oral Medicine, Oral Pathology,* 73(1992): 139.
Data in the table is based on the *WHO Weekly
Epidemiological Record,* No. 40, October 5, 1990.

(rate per million) for selected countries. The data in this table and in Table 5–2 indicate that Cuba has one of the lowest AIDS incidence rates in the world. In April 1991, Dr. Hector Terry and Dr. Francisco Machado reported that the infection rate for all of Cuba is .06 percent. (9,771,691 tested; total population is over 10,000,000.)[32] Although I am critical of the HIV quarantine, a major feature of Cuban policy, the facts in Tables 5–1 and 5–2 are straightforward: Cuba has kept the AIDS epidemic under control and contained the spread of AIDS.

For patients in a hospital or a prenatal clinic, or anywhere else where blood samples are taken and tested, the test for HIV is now one of the routine tests done in Cuba. Most people are probably not aware that their blood is being tested for the virus. Those who are screened in residential settings or at the workplace are aware only when the process is for the specific purpose of testing for the HIV virus. There have been reports of some people refusing to be tested.[33] These people are not forced to give a blood sample, but a great deal of peer pressure is put on them to do so from the mass organizations, the block committees, their family doctors and coworkers who believe strongly that cooperation with the testing program is for the common good.

Testing is supervised and checked by a national laboratory, although the administration and processing of the tests are carried out at the provincial level. If a sample tests positive, two or three additional tests are done to confirm the results. "Persons with borderline results are followed in the community under very strict confidentiality, providing them with intensive counseling and support, until a definitive diagnosis is reached."[34]

Research studies in the United States on the rate of false positives in test procedures for HIV infection suggest that the data presented in Table 5–1 in all probability include false positives. Ronald Bayer and Cheryl Healton of the Columbia University School of Public Health believe they do: "With infection rates of .01 percent or less, even when stringent laboratory standards are maintained, one in 135,000 would be mistakenly designated as positive. More typical laboratory standards would produce much higher false positive rates. We estimate that among the seven low-infection groups tested in Cuba, between 21 and 53 persons may have been inaccurately considered positive as a result of testing."[35]

When Dr. Francisco Machado, head of Cuba's national laboratory conducting research on AIDS, was asked about the unjust quarantine of people, he responded, "I can publicly assure you that not a single person is unjustly quarantined in Cuba."[36] The reason he could be so categorical, he explained, was because in the last analysis of whether the diagnosis is negative, positive, or indeterminate, "we follow the criteria of the Center for Disease Control in Atlanta, Georgia, because we consider them as the best in the world."[37] . . .

Public Fear and Ignorance

AIDS is not just an epidemic; it is also a social and political phenomenon. How an epidemic is understood in social and political terms, in turn, affects the disease's progress and its medical treatment. Thus, diseases are never simply medical problems. Epidemics, in particular, become the focus of social attitudes because they raise the spector of mass death.

In 1988 an article on AIDS in *Cuba International* began:

> Some months ago, the Buenos Aires magazine *Somos* told the story of an Argentine entrepreneur who went on a business trip to Brazil and who decided, before returning, to have a wild weekend. When he awoke on Monday morning he found the girl he had spent the past two nights with gone. On the bathroom mirror he read with horror the following words written in lipstick: "Congratulations, you have just joined the AIDS brigade."
>
> Around the same time, the Madrid magazine *Tiempo* described in graphic detail the death of Tarim, a homosexual and make-up artist who had been a darling of the jet set.
>
> A Spanish writer, Sánchez Ocana, in his book *What Can I Do About AIDS?* has a whole chapter on the problems of homosexuality and drug addiction in Spanish jails, and says that the prison authorities now distribute condoms and hypodermic needles among the inmates to protect them from AIDS.
>
> Acquired Immune Deficiency Syndrome (AIDS) is both an individual and a collective issue. Thousands of scientists around the world are concentrating their energies on finding a cure for it. A U.S. doctor compared it to the "black plague" that killed a third of Europe's population in the 14th century.[38]

These few introductory paragraphs illustrate age-old attitudes common to many societies and many epidemics: that the disease is brought in by foreigners, that it is caused by moral corruption, that if no salvation is found total destruction will result.

Robert Swenson, an infectious disease specialist and immunologist with an interest in the history of epidemics, analyzed AIDS and other plagues in history with reference to what he calls the "internal anatomy of an epidemic"—that is, attitudes and behavior.[39] One of these identified attitudes is to place blame elsewhere for the epidemic.

> Once the epidemic is recognized, it follows quickly that someone (something else) is blamed for it. As the bubonic plague swept through Europe in 1348, it was claimed that it was caused by Jews who had poisoned wells. As a result, thousands of Jews were burned at the stake. The cholera epidemics in the United States fell disproportionately on the poor. At that time, poverty was viewed as a consequence of idleness and intemperance. The latter was also clearly felt to make one more susceptible to cholera. Since new immigrants were often the most poor, they were blamed for their own susceptibility to cholera, as well as for bringing the disease into the country. Prostitutes were also blamed for the epidemic, even though cholera was not thought to be a venereal disease. Many felt that their "moral corruption" caused them, as well as their clients, to develop cholera.
>
> Blame would also be placed at a national level. After the initial outbreak of influenza in the United States, epidemics occurred in Spain, England, and France. In addition to attempting to deny their own epidemics, the countries blamed one another. The French referred to the epidemic as the Plague of the Spanish Lady, and the English called it the French Disease. (Even today we refer to the Asian Flu.)[40]

Fidel Castro himself followed this tradition in a September 1988 speech: "Who brought AIDS to Latin America? Who was the great AIDS vector in the Third World? Why are there countries like the Dominican Republic, with 40,000 carriers of the virus; and Haiti, and other countries of Central America and South America—high rates in Mexico, in Brazil and other countries? Who brought it? The United States, that's a fact."[41]

The foreign power that had militarily invaded Cuba in the past, that had made numerous assassination attempts on his life, that maintained hostile policies, could now easily be blamed for introducing the plague. This sense of an island under siege no doubt has contributed to the decision to control the disease through the drastic means of a quarantine.

The quarantine policy itself has contributed to the popular panic about AIDS. People feel, "We are all safe, as long as they are kept behind the sanitorium walls," and thus they support the quarantine policy. For example, when Alfaro Mendoza, a twenty-six-year-old graduate student, was told by his doctors that he should go to the sanitorium, a friend of his agreed: "It's too bad for him, but he got infected, and it's safer for everybody that he go; and it's safer for us."[42] Monika Krause notes that sanitorium isolation makes minimal educational campaigns even more difficult because the population now feels safe and no longer takes the threat of AIDS seriously.[43]

There is general ignorance about the difference between someone with AIDS and someone who has tested HIV–positive but is nevertheless a healthy person, who may never become ill with an AIDS–related disease. The quarantine does nothing to diminish this ignorance; in fact, the press often refers to sanitorium residents as "AIDS patients"—a phenomenon Susan Sontag has observed in the United States.

> The obvious consequence of believing that all those who "harbor" the virus will eventually come down with the illness is that those who test positive for it are regarded as people-with-AIDS, who just don't have it . . . yet. It is only a matter of time, like any death sentence. Less obviously, such people are often regarded as if they do have it. Testing positive for HIV, which usually means having been tested for the presence not of the virus but of antibodies to the virus, is increasingly being equated with being ill.[44]

Machismo, the "Uncontrollable Force"

Two assumptions dominate the Cuban quarantine policy: First, people will always be irresponsible in terms of sex, and no policy of safe sex will work that relies on individual control. Second, education cannot change this behavior. Since, therefore, it is impossible to know which infected people can be trusted to behave responsibly, all must be treated as dangerous.

Both assumptions are rooted in macho mentality and have long been a barrier to controlling sexually transmitted diseases. Referring to nineteenth century England and venereal disease, Robert Swenson wrote:

> With the realization that these were sexually transmitted diseases with grave health consequences (mental illness and infertility, for example), it was recognized that there was a need for sex education; yet great obstacles existed to what became known as the social hygiene movement. First, the remaining tenets of Victorian respectability made it virtually impossible to discuss venereal diseases. The basic assumption was that men were driven by lust and that discussing sex with them would only make them more uncontrollable. The major question became, how can sex education be presented to men without their recognizing the subject? The answer was to include much talk about the plants, birds, bees, and little about sex. Given these subterfuges, there could be little effective sex education. Prince Morrow, a leader of the social hygiene movement, concluded, "Social sentiment holds that it is a greater violation of the properties of life publicly to mention venereal disease than privately to contract it."[45]

The idea that the male sexual urge is uncontrollable is shared by women, as well, where it prevails. This is why, in many societies, it has been the custom that an unmarried woman should never be alone with a man as he could not be expected to control himself. Speaking of a Cuban friend living in the Havana sanitorium, Bill Rowe, who served on the Emergency AIDS Task Force for the American Anthropological Association, discovered similar attitudes in Cuba regarding uncontrollable male sexual urges. His friend had tested HIV–positive but had no symptoms and reported "no negative health conditions." He was chaperoned by a medical student during his regular Sunday visits home. After speaking to the man's family and friends, Rowe reported that "the elderly ex-banker, heterosexual father of the household, his gay son, and his gay son's lover, all explained to me very forcefully that Cuban men would require that kind of chaperonage. That male sexuality was a totally uncontrollable force."[46]

Both the acceptance of irresponsible sex as a social norm and the limitations of the quarantine policy are painfully evident in interviews with some of the people confined to the sanitorium. A young man who is confined in the sanitorium, shares his experience.

> I think that the isolation is dreadful. It's dreadful. I understand it. There are cases where really I understand it because not everybody has "conciencia." I say that, together with HIV, comes a heavy responsibility. There are people who simply do not have this "conciencia" and are really dangerous. I don't know; I have no idea how to solve this. I think it's difficult, but there must be a solution because we can't stay here all our lives. And besides, nobody knows when people will get it, and so they can't spend their lives here. For example, the people who may live 10, 20 years . . . (Raúl, a resident in the Havana sanitorium, 1989)[47]

The assumption that male sexual behavior is unchangeable makes the quarantine policy, with its reliance on testing, seem the only solution. However, not only is it based on a false assumption about the accuracy of the "testing net," but recent research indicates new medical treatments that delay AIDS even further . . .[48]

Cuba's Authoritarian Government

Visitors to the Cuban sanitoriums report seeing healthy-looking people—in most cases asymptomatic—in a confined residence, not working at their trained occupation but "serving time," no matter how "pleasant" the surroundings. One report in *Granma* on the Havana sanitorium showed a picture of a man and woman walking on a road with the caption: "It's difficult to tell patients from workers because most seem strong and healthy."[49] But one of the "patients" revealed the difference.

> At first it was rough; they didn't tell me I was sick until I got here. Now it's better. I share this house with my wife and work in the carpentry and refrigeration department when I feel like it. What I want most is for time to pass so I can go home (about 160 kilometers from Havana). I have nothing to complain about concerning the way I'm treated. There are a lot of people from my home town who joke and say I'm not sick, that I'm living off the government.[50]

The workers can go home at night. They have control over their own lives denied to the "patients." The possibility of the residents doing some kind of work within the sanitorium was one of the reforms instituted at Los Cocos by the new director who took over in early 1989. For four of the residents who are doctors, it meant they could at least continue to practice medicine within the sanitorium. One of them expressed what a vast improvement that was:

> Something else I saw in the director, and it's very important. He believes in people. He believes in us. . . . One of the things I observed was that, from the moment we had AIDS (sic), we became "irresponsible" people, people who had no reason to be . . . we were completely nullified socially, intellectually; and he, he believes in us and gives us opportunities to grow, to do something useful. . . . when he called me to talk and see if I would like to work, I asked, "Is it true?" . . . at first I endeavored to see if it were true, if I really was going to be a doctor in this institution. They simply showed me that, yes, I have my own patients; I have everything, and I work as a doctor.
>
> Now, the only thing that's missing is to demonstrate that we have "conciencia," that we are normal people equal to everyone else, that we can work, that we can lead a social life like other people and conduct ourselves as we have and as many people in the streets who don't have AIDS do.[51]

The physician, Juan Carlos, also prepared a written statement on the quarantine policy, parts of which I reproduce below. (Omitted are descriptions already incorporated in this chapter.) Following the statement is a transcript of part of a conversation between Juan Carlos and another young man confined to the sanitorium. The contrast is revealing. The statement is very careful and does not question policies. Not that he does not believe what he is writing, but unlike the conversation, his writing does not reflect his real anguish and awareness that an alternative is possible.

> There is a great difference between the sanitorium's past and present from the point of view of isolation. At the beginning, we found ourselves almost totally isolated from society because the visits from relatives were restricted, because the means of transmission were not completely known. This isolation lasted a few months, and a system of passes and structured leaves was established and perfected over time.
>
> We must take into account that the population of the sanitorium is heterogeneous and constitutes a micro-society in which there are people fully aware of the situation—who feel a tremendous social responsibility. But, on the other hand, it is certain that we don't all think alike, and that is why any patient leaving the sanitorium is accompanied by health department personnel who will prevent sexual contact and foresee any possible incident. With experience, it has been decided to attempt to modify this system of leaves, taking into account individual character and the degree of social responsibility acquired for each one of the patients.
>
> Inside the sanitorium, all the conditions exist to make possible a restful life. Participation in sports and adequate nutrition are provided. We go to the beach and the movies regularly as well as museums and recreational centers. But, of course, admission to the sanitorium is a radical change in our lives and in one aspect that I consider fundamental: It cuts us off from work. Although we can fill the free time with other activities, it just leaves a vacuum and longing for the work we were trained for. At present, this is a concern for everybody—patients,

MINSAP, the government. There is an attempt at connecting patients with work so we can feel socially useful.

I must also say that the stay in the sanitorium permits better medical care, and I must emphasize that this is the only country in the world where detected HIV carriers are checked regularly whether they are healthy or sick. This makes greater survival possible. I think that, with the little I have explained, you can get a brief idea of our sanitorium from its beginnings—how it evolved in its efforts to improve and achieve its goal with a more humane perspective. In a certain way, it has protected us from rejection from society when it was believed that AIDS was a disease afflicting only homosexual and drug addicts or, to be more precise, people with an incorrect social conduct.[52]

Juan Carlos and his friend Raúl both advocate treating the problem of AIDS and HIV by keeping certain aspects of the sanitorium system, specifically as a center for HIV checkups and medical treatment of HIV–positive people. But they also want those who test HIV–positive to be treated with the same dignity as other people. They want to live normally. In this conversation, they debate the question of their rights and the ability of patients to leave the sanitorium—the problem of those who are irresponsible and therefore "dangerous to others":

Raúl: This behavior today (forming couples, avoiding bathrooms, etc.) is intelligent, and they must also contact the sanitorium to get treatment. But they must also be integrated into society, like a diabetic who works everyday, like someone with high blood pressure, like—I don't know—like any sick person, sensibly and simply.

I would agree that we are here for medical care . . . but for me, on the human aspect I also think we need to be outside, go to the movies, and do other things. Do you want to have a mark on a part of your body?

Juan: But why not? Look, I was thinking . . .

Rául: So we can be outside and be free?

Juan: At some point I thought: "Look, put on my I.D. that I am an HIV CARRIER."

Rául: No, Chico, that's useless.

Juan: Wait a minute, let me explain. I would prefer to have a really big placard in front of me saying: "HIV POSITIVE" and be on the street than be confined. I don't care if I have AIDS and that people know that I have AIDS and want to look at me or not. I don't care about that because the people I'm interested in treat me according to my politics, my personality.

But my great anger is about all this effort I made to develop a career and that all of that was suddenly, completely destroyed. I have not been able to develop myself socially. If they want me to wear a big poster, right here in front. . . .

It seems to me that you're exaggerating a little . . . there are people who will never be able to leave this place. It's the same as the thief that spends his life stealing and, therefore, must be kept in jail. Please, that's evident. It's evident. It's his way.

Moreover, when you sit down to talk with people here, you can classify all those who should not leave this place. You're sure that they have to stay here. Unfortunately, it has to be so. If they're not here, they're going to be put in jail or be locked up somewhere else. You have to understand, they are people who socially contribute nothing. . . . there's something else. Here there are many people whom I think . . . it is a question of a psychological approach . . . who just are not responsible, who think they are not sick, that they're not dangerous. But if these people were persuaded, were made sensitive to the problem they have, then I think they could be outside.[53]

Providing the possibility for work within the sanitorium was certainly an important advance in the patient's quality of life. Apparently there has been some further reform. Dr. Hector Terry was quoted in a *Granma International* article saying, "Several of our hospitalized AIDS patients go to their jobs daily and sleep in the sanitorium. As time goes by, the restrictions could become more flexible, but it will all depend on how responsible each patient proves to be. I reiterate that our responsibility as the government is to protect all citizens."[54]

But most of the 703 people confined to a sanitorium do not have the possibility of meaningful work and cannot go out to jobs. No matter how much institutional life is cloaked with a "children's camp" style of recreational activities, such as trips to the beach and the movies, the basic condition of life is confinement and enforced passivity—waiting for death or the Big Cure, being "saved by world science," in Dr. Terry's words. The extensive health care that prolongs the lives of people carrying HIV is commendable, but these are basically healthy people who are being treated by the medical establishment as though they were sick—patients who cannot be expected to exercise any control over their lives. Those who have succumbed to opportunistic cancers and infections because of their immune deficiency are certainly patients, but being the carrier of a virus does not make one so. Yet Dr. Terry himself refers to residents of a sanitorium, who have only tested HIV–positive, as "hospitalized AIDS patients."

Cuban government spokesmen perpetuate the myth that "there is no other alternative to quarantine." However, there is an alternative. Dr. Jonathan Mann, former director of the World Health Organization's program on AIDS said when asked about the Cuban quarantine program: "We don't think well of it. In fact, the World Health Organization has very strong policies, including a resolution passed by the latest world health assembly, that specifically state that discrimination against people who are infected should not be allowed . . . people lose confidence in the ability to educate and would rather have confidence in laws or in jails."[55]

In July 1989, at a meeting sponsored by WHO and the UN Commission on Human Rights, H. Daniel, a Brazilian revolutionary who spent seven years in political exile, made public a letter he had written to Fidel Castro. As a follower of Che Guevara and a person with AIDS, Daniel wrote that there were no possible arguments to defend Cuba's quarantine policies "except for those based on the most reactionary forms of prejudice against gays" that will, in the end, be "counterproductive." In his letter, he spoke first of Brazil, where,

> From the beginning, the AIDS epidemic was not taken seriously by our authorities. And, up to this day, there is nothing close to a national program to control the epidemic and assist those with AIDS, even though Brazil is one of the countries most affected by this illness in the world. Beyond this, old prejudices against gays are added to the new stigmas that mark this recent global epidemic, stigmas which marginalize the person with AIDS. Deprived of basic human rights, the person with AIDS experiences a de facto civil death.

H. Daniel then contrasted that with Cuba:

> I have followed with great sorrow the Cuban initiatives in relation to AIDS. From Cuba especially, I hoped for a great example in the search for solutions to this very grave public health problem. Cuba could take pride in its health system. Could, if it weren't for the way it treats those who are HIV seropositive, whether sick or not, burying them in an isolation which has no technical justification, which goes against all scientific advice and which seriously infringes on human rights.
>
> Cuba has used, in an abusive manner, compulsory HIV tests and has incarcerated those who test positively. Thus Cuba seeks to combat the virus by combating those people whom the virus attacked. In this way, Cuba is defeated by the HIV virus and by the ideological virus of prejudice and discrimination. There are no possible arguments to defend these positions, except for those based on the most reactionary forms of prejudice against gays.
>
> Certainly Cuba will soon discover that these measures are counterproductive. People with AIDS will be placed in the position of enemies, even more difficult to locate, and the epidemic will *not* be overcome. The only result will be to impose absurd suffering on those who today could easily contribute to control of the epidemic, as has been happening in other countries of the world.

Daniel concludes his letter with a plea:

> In my name, in the name of the 10 million people with AIDS across the world, of their families and friends, in the name of all who believe in life as an act of freedom, I ask you, compañero Fidel, to change the Cuban AIDS program. First, it is necessary to free those political prisoners. Second, it is necessary to implement a program based on the revolutionary principle of solidarity.
>
> I sincerely hope that Cuba will not permit itself to be defeated by prejudice.
>
> H. Daniel
> Rio de Janeiro, Brazil[56]

The experience of people with AIDS in Brazil and many other countries is similar to that in the United States. Douglas Crimp expresses it so well:

> Most people dying of AIDS are very young, and those of us coping with these deaths, ourselves also young, have confronted great loss entirely unprepared. The number of deaths are unthinkable: lovers, friends, acquaintances, and com-

munity members have fallen ill and died. Many have lost upwards of a hundred people. . . .

Through the turmoil imposed by illness and death, the rest of society offers little support or even acknowledgment. On the contrary, we are blamed, belittled, excluded, derided. We are discriminated against, we lose our housing and jobs and are denied medical and life insurance. Every public agency whose job it is to combat the epidemic has been slow to act, failed entirely, or been deliberately counterproductive. We have therefore had to provide our own centers for support, care, and education, and even fund our own treatment research. We have had to rebuild our devastated community and culture, reconstruct our sexual relationships, reinvent our sexual pleasure.[57]

In the United States the fight is against not only the sex and racial prejudices of society, but a government whose policies demonstrate deep disregard for those on the bottom. Thus, the Cuban officials argue that their policy is more just for all. When Vice-Minister Terry was asked about Cuba's position on human rights and AIDS, he defended it and juxtaposed the United States' neglect of people with AIDS:

To respond to this question, it seems very important to define our concepts of discrimination, exclusion, and human rights. . . .

In Cuba, nobody lacks economic resources because of being an AIDS carrier. In Cuba, no one dies abandoned on the streets for lack of access to a hospital. In Cuba, we haven't had to open hospices so that patients who have been abandoned have a place to die in peace. In Cuba, no one's house has been set on fire because its inhabitants are people with AIDS. In Cuba, no homosexual has been persecuted because he's assumed to be likely to spread the virus. In Cuba, we don't have the problem of national minorities or drug addicts with high rates of AIDS.

Our country has more than 10 million inhabitants, all of whom are guaranteed the right to health care, and that is why the immense majority of the population backs the AIDS prevention and Control program. Therefore, our concept of human rights is in no way incompatible with that of the WHO. We are convinced that we are respecting the rights of those who are ill with AIDS or carrying the virus, and we are protecting the rights of the immerse majority of the population that is still healthy.[58]

The Cuban government claims great success for its quarantine policy—"the proportion of carriers to patients is 5.4 to 1, as compared to an estimated 60–100 to 1 in countries where no checks exist"[59]—and proudly acknowledges that the country stands alone with its AIDS policy.

No other country in the world is concerned with checking its seropositive patients. This is so because other countries are either unable to do it from the practical point of view or for economic or social reasons. The fact is that they don't know who the seropositive cases are and so the figures they report are estimates based on studies of representative groups. . . . As a result, no direct action is being taken to avoid the sexual transmission of the disease that, as we know, is the most common means and the one responsible for the pandemic dissemination the virus has acquired. The strategy of isolating patients and carriers under a sanitorium regime is justified from the epidemiological point of view, provided that it is possible to detect most of the cases; otherwise, the effect this would have on the sexual transmission of the HIV would be cancelled out by transmission among undetected cases.

The main usefulness of this measure is to slow down the epidemic progression of the disease to allow time for other measures of disease control to have a medium- or long-time effect.[60]

Four years later, on December 1, 1992, Dr. Terry underscored again that the six-year-old quarantine policy "has protected the vast majority of the Cuban people, including those with AIDS." The director of the AIDS Advice and Information Center in Havana, Dr. Giselle Sanabria, reported that 98 percent of the HIV–positive persons (the 703 people in the sanitoriums) contracted the virus through sexual relations. 41 percent were homosexual or bisexual while 57 percent were heterosexual. The other 2 percent were infected by blood transfusions, most of them in 1986 before the introduction of careful controls. There are no reports of any drug related cases.[61]

In their rush to quarantine, the Cubas have edited out one important, but crucial, point: *it is possible to prevent new infections.* Unlike epidemics in earlier historical periods, *we do know how AIDS is transmitted.* These behaviors are identifiable and recognizable. Because of this, it is possible to prevent the spread of the virus. It requires information and education programs in all countries.[62]

However, in most countries, including Cuba, the taboo subject of sexual practices—especially homosexual ones—is part of old inhibitions that have not been shed. The minimalist Cuban AIDS educational campaign is aimed entirely at heterosexuals and ignores the increase in HIV infections among homosexuals. Of course, behavioral change through education is not easy, especially when education means little more than advertising campaigns and catchy slogans. A follow-up study on one such campaign in the United States indicated that 60 percent of those originally influenced by the advertisements only occasionally used a condom.[63]

NOTES

1. Some people call AIDS "full blown AIDS"; in this text *HIV positive* will be used for people who have tested positive for the HIV virus. It is not only redundant to use language like "full blown AIDS" but such language implies that HIV positive tested people have AIDS, which is not true. If they come down with AIDS, then they will be people with AIDS.

2. *Primer Seminario Sobre Infección Por VIH y SIDA en Cuba, Octubre 30 y 31, 1992: Libro de Resumenes* (Havana: Sanitario Santiago de Las Vegas, Ministerio de Salud Pública, 1992), 1; Reuters International Dispatch (Havana: Reuters, 14:42, December 1, 1992); Dr. Hector Terry, Vice-Minister of Public Health, *Radio Havana Report on AIDS in Cuba*, February 28, 1993.

Also see: Carlos Cabrera, "Fight against Death," *International Granma*, April 7, 1991, 8. This is one of the lowest AIDS infection rates in the world and the lowest in Latin America. *Newsday*, "Cuba's AIDS Success," April 10, 1991; Robert Collier, "AIDS: Cuba's Quarantine," *Newsday*, May 2, 1989, Discovery section, 3; also see Ronald Bayer and Cheryl Healton, Special Report: "Controlling AIDS in Cuba: The Logic of the Quarantine," *The New England Journal of Medicine*, April 13, 1989, 1022–1024; Sarah Santana, "AIDS in Cuba," *Cuba Update*, Summer 1989: 23–25.

3. The Cuban Ministry of Health states that the special treatment and diets have extended the average survival rate to seven years. Dr. Hector Terry, public health deputy minister, as quoted in Carlos Cabrera, "Fight Against Death," 8; see Gina Kolata, "Studies Cite 10.5 Years From Infection to Illness," *New York Times*, November 8, 1991, B12.

4. "The AIDS Battle: Tempered by Experience," *Cuba Update*, Summer 1991: 23–24.

5. Bayer and Healton, "Controlling AIDS," 1023; Santana, "AIDS in Cuba," 23.

6. Carlos Cabrera, "On the Frontiers of AIDS," *Weekly Granma*, December 10, 1989, 12.

7. Interview with Cuban Ministry of Health (MINSAP) officials, February 1988.

8. Cabrera, "On the Frontiers of AIDS," 12.

9. Karen Wald, "Cuban Health Official Talks About AIDS Policy," *Cuba Update*, Summer 1989: 26.

10. Karen Wald, "Questions and Answers on AIDS in Cuba," (unpublished interview with Dr. Hector Terry, 1989).

11. Bayer and Healton, "Controlling AIDS," 1023; MINSAP, February 1988 interview; Cabrera, "On the Frontiers of AIDS," 12.

12. Santana, "AIDS in Cuba," 24. It appears very few people have earned this special privilege; for summaries of scientific papers presented at the October 1992 Havana "First Seminar on HIV Infections and AIDS in Cuba" see *Primer Seminario Sobre Infección Por VIH*, 1–45; see Robert Bazell, "Happy Campers," *The New Republic*, March 9, 1992, 12, 14.

In June, 1993 the Cuban government announced a further easing of its quarantine policy. After six months of quarantine and "political education" individuals deemed trustworthy will be allowed to live "freely as long as they behave properly." Those who cannot qualify will continue to stay in the sanitorium with weekend passes by chaperone "until they modify their conduct." Radio Havana Cuba, "Cuba's New AIDS Policy," June 21, 1993; Laurie Garrett, "Cuba Institutes a Freer AIDS Policy," *New York Newsday*, August 3, 1993, 53, 59.

13. "The AIDS Battle," *Cuba Update*, Summer 1991: 23–24; Garrett, "Cuba Institutes Freer AIDS Policy," 59.

14. Cabrera, "On the Frontiers of AIDS," 12.

15. *Sideroso:* a term taken from the Spanish word for AIDS—Sida.

16. Karen Wald, "Visits to the Sanitorium" (Los Cocos, Havana; unpublished interviews, July 1989).

17. Santana, "AIDS in Cuba," 23.

18. Ministry of Health Officials (MINSAP) interview, February 1988.

19. Ministry of Health (MINSAP) interview, 1988.

20. Cabrera, "On the Frontiers of AIDS," 12.

21. Hector Terry in Wald, "Questions and Answers."

22. Margaret Gilpin, "Cuba: On the Road to a Family Medicine NATION," *Family Medicine* 21 (November–December 1989): 405; Robert Ubell, "High Tech Medicine in the Caribbean," *New England Journal of Medicine* 309 (December 1983): 1468; Julie Feinsilver, "Cuba As a 'World Medical Power': The Politics of Symbolism," *Latin American Research Review* 24 (1989): 1–33.

23. Harry Nelson, "Overmedicated?: An Excess of Success May Ail Cuba's Top-Flight Health Care System," *Cuba Update,* November 1991: 33–34 (originally published in *Los Angeles Times,* July 22, 1991); also see Feinsilver, "Cuba As A World Medical Power."

24. Jeanne Smith and Sergio Piomelli, "Letters: The War on AIDS," *New York Times,* January 22, 1989, 24E.

25. Sarah Santana, "AIDS in Cuba: The AIDS Program," *Cuba Update,* Summer 1989: 23.

26. Paula A. Treichler, "AIDS and HIV Infection in the Third World: A First World Chronicle," in Elizabeth Fee and Daniel M. Fox, eds., *AIDS: The Making of a Chronic Disease* (Berkeley: University of California Press, 1992), 392; see also Hector Terry in Wald, "Questions and Answers"; see also Elizabeth Fee, "Sex Education in Cuba: An Interview With Dr. Celestino Lajonchere," *International Journal of Health Services,* 18, no. 2 (1988), 343–56; Nicholas Wade, "Cuba's Quarantine For AIDS: A Police State's Health Experiment," *New York Times,* editorial, February 6, 1989, A14.

27. Bruce Lambert, "The Best AIDS Programs Are Too Few for Too Many," *New York Times,* June 15, 1990, B4.

28. Carlos Cabrera, "AIDS: Fight Against Death," *International Granma,* April 7, 1991, 8.

29. Marlise Simons, "A Latin AIDS Meeting Opens its Ears to What Was Once Unmentionable," *New York Times,* January 16, 1989, A6; Collier, "Cuba's Quarantine," 3.

30. Santana, "AIDS in Cuba," 23.

31. Karen Wald, "AIDS in Cuba: A Dream or a Nightmare?" *Z Magazine,* December 1990, 104–109.

32. Carlos Cabrera, "Fight Against Death," 8; Dr. Abelardo Martínez, Prof. Hector de Arazoza, Dr. José Joanes, Dr. Rigoberto Torres, Dr. Jorge Pérez, *"Comportamiento del SIDA en Cuba Hasta 30–de Septiembre, 1992,"* in *Primer Seminario Sobre Infección por VIH y SIDA en Cuba,* 1.

33. Santana, "AIDS in Cuba," 23.

34. Ibid.

35. Bayer and Healton, "Controlling AIDS in Cuba," 1023.

36. Cabrera, "Fight Against Death," 8.

37. The respect for the capacity of the United States to offer high standards in technology and the sciences went beyond Dr. Machado's statement about the Center for Disease Control being the "best in the world." In spite of the blockade, but with much hardship (sometimes getting materials via Canada and Europe) Cuban educators did learn about some of the curriculum changes in U.S. public schools. For example, I was surprised in 1969 when I interviewed Dr. María de Carmen Nuñoz Berro. In charge of introducing a modern mathematics program from kindergarten through senior high school, she was familiar with and favorably impressed by such U.S. mathematics programs as the Greater Cleveland Program and the Madison Program. And, as indicated earlier, the sex educators in GNTES were familiar and articulate about John Money, Helen Singer Kaplan, and other U.S. experts on sex education.

38. Ciro Bianchi Ross, "To Contain AIDS," *Cuba International,* January 1988, 8.

39. Robert Swenson, "Plagues, History, and AIDS," *The American Scholar* 57 (Spring 1988): 188.

40. Ibid.

41. Fidel speech in *Granma,* September 1988.

42. Collier, "Cuba's Quarantine," 3; Dr. Hector Terry, Vice Minister of Public Health "admitted that AIDS education has been one of weakest links in the island's AIDS program. There is still much to be done, he said, to get the message across to people by making more effective use of the mass media." Dr. Hector Terry, *Radio Havana Report on AIDS,* February 28, 1993.

43. Wald, "A Dream or a Nightmare," 106.

44. Susan Sontag, *AIDS and Its Metaphors* (New York: Farrar, Strauss and Giroux, 1989), 32.

45. Swenson, "Plagues, History and AIDS," 189.

46. Karen Wald, "Interview with Bill Rowe, National AIDS Task Force of the American Anthropological Association," September 1988.

47. Karen Wald, "Conversations in Sanitorium" (Los Cocos, Havana; unpublished interviews, September 1989).

48. Philip J. Hilts, "Drug Said To Help AIDS Cases With Virus But No Symptoms," *New York Times,* August 18, 1989, A1.

49. Cabrera, "On the Frontiers of AIDS," 12.

50. Ibid.

51. Wald, "Conversations in Sanitorium."

52. Ibid.

53. Ibid.

54. Dr. Hector Terry as quoted in Cabrera, "Fight Against Death," 8.

55. Jonathan Mann, in interview on PBS' AIDS Quarterly, April 25, interviewed by Peter Jennings.

56. "Letters: AIDS in Cuba," *New York Review of Books,* October 26, 1989, 68–69.

57. Douglas Crimp, "Mourning and Militancy," *October* 51 (Winter 1989): 15.

58. Hector Terry in Wald, "Questions and Answers."

59. Editorial, "Cuban Strategy in the Struggle Against AIDS," *Weekly Granma,* September 18, 1988.

60. Ibid.

61. Reuters International Dispatch, December 1, 1992; Bazell, "Happy Camper," 14. Recent reports from health officials on the AIDS epidemic in Latin America indicate an alarming increase in the rate of HIV infection and AIDS. Cuba is the one exception in the region. "Latin America's most successful effort in limiting the spread of the infection has apparently been in Cuba," James Brooke, "In Deception and Denial, an Epidemic Looms," *New York Times,* January 25, 1993, A6.

62. Mann, "The International Epidemiology of AIDS," 89.

63. Harvey V. Fineberg, "The Social Dimensions of AIDS," *Scientific American* 259, no. 4 (October 1988): 130; Bazell, "Happy Camper," 14.

11

The International Response

Yole G. Sills

Any assessment of the social consequences of the AIDS pandemic must include its extraordinary impact on international relations. The fear and in some cases the panic engendered by AIDS have triggered two dramatically different reactions. The first has been a negative, defensive reaction expressed by governments and by hostile press and media coverage that threatened to sour international relations—particularly in the first years of the AIDS pandemic. The second, in marked contrast, is an overwhelmingly positive, unprecedented cooperative global effort to combat the epidemic.

XENOPHOBIC REACTIONS TO AIDS

More than fifty countries all over the world have imposed exclusionary restrictions on the international travel and immigration of people with HIV and AIDS, ranging from tourism to business travel, to immigration, to student exchanges (Tomasevski 1992:555). Belgium, Bulgaria, Czechoslovakia, Costa Rica, Cuba, France, Hungary, Iraq, Kuwait, Saudi Arabia, South Korea, the former Soviet Union, Sweden, Thailand, the United Arab Emirates, and the United States are among the countries that already employ mandatory testing of blood for all but short-term visitors. Reactions to AIDS in sub–Saharan

Sills, Yole G. "The International Response," from *The AIDS Pandemic* (London: Greenwood Press, 1994), pp. 99–119. Reprinted by permission of Greenwood Publishing Group, Inc., Westport, CT.

African countries have been similar to those in Europe and North America—with compulsory screening of both immigrants and entering students (Krisber & Blaney 1987). Algeria, Morocco, and Syria, on the other hand, test the blood of all returning nationals.

The Indian Council of Medical Research has proposed that sex relations with an infected foreigner be made a criminal offense punishable by a fine or a prison sentence. Foreign students cannot enroll in Indian universities without HIV clearance certificates and visitors who want to stay in India for more than three months are subjected to mandatory testing (Misztal & Moss 1990: 10). China limits contacts between its citizens and foreigners. In South Africa, migrant workers from neighboring states who are found to be HIV positive are deported. In Japan, which has had relatively few cases but which is experiencing an increase, a prevention campaign poster urges caution while traveling abroad by depicting a man carrying his passport—indicating that the danger is in catching the disease while away from Japan (*New York Times*, November 8, 1992:13).

In the United States, infection with HIV is one of the conditions that can bar entry to immigrants, refugees, and visitors (unless visitors can obtain a waiver). This policy has been fraught with controversy and has been repeatedly criticized by public health experts within the government, as well as by numerous AIDS advocacy organizations, as being needlessly discriminatory. The reality is that some 1 million people in the United States are already infected with HIV. In January 1991, Louis Sullivan, the U.S. secretary of health and human services, proposed that aliens with HIV not be excluded from the United States because they would not pose a significant additional risk of HIV infection to the U.S. population, since AIDS cannot be transmitted by casual contact (*New York Times*, January 4, 1991:A1, A15).

Publication of the Sullivan proposal in the *Federal Register* raised a storm of protest in the Congress as well as from conservative groups all over the country. Representative William E. Dannemeyer, Republican of California, attacked the proposal as being inconsistent: "On the one hand they say AIDS is a major problem; on the other hand, they say we should take in AIDS carriers with impunity." Others objected that allowing infected aliens to enter would expose the country to potentially huge medical costs. The issue was debated for the next two years by both the public and the Congress. Finally, on March 11, 1993, the House of Representatives followed an earlier vote in the Senate and voted "to ban immigration into the United States by people infected with the virus that causes AIDS" (*New York Times*, March 12, 1993: A11).[1]

As in the case of such diseases as syphilis and smallpox, other countries, generally the United States or the countries of sub–Saharan Africa, are often blamed for AIDS. In France, as Dennis Altman (1986) observed, AIDS was at least initially seen as an American import. In the United Kingdom, AIDS has been blamed on homosexuals who have been on sex holidays to America.

Dorothy Nelkin and Sander L. Gilman reported that the French labeled AIDS an "American disease" as early as 1981, referring to the American influence on French attitudes toward homosexuality. For some segments of the French public, they noted, "AIDS was but another example of the American corruption of the French body politic, but now in the form of a 'real disease.' " Amyl nitrate "poppers," used to enhance sexual experience during homosexual acts, were labeled "an American pollutant consumed here." The French government warned the gay "jet set" that it was at risk because of the "American connection" (Nelkin & Gilman 1988:364).

In India, consorting with foreigners is the focus of blame. In a lead story in the weekly magazine *Sunday*, A. S. Paintal (1989), director of the Indian Council of Medical Research, declared "AIDS is being poured into women. If women (prostitutes) had taken steps two years ago and stopped cohabiting with foreigners, then the situation would not have become so dangerous." In the Philippines, suspicions that American military personnel were potential carriers of AIDS to the local population became part of the discussions concerning the renewal of American bases and provoked angry polemics in Japan (Ergas 1987).[2]

The "blame the foreigner" syndrome has been most in evidence in the widely reported series of accusatory exchanges that have characterized the reciprocal attitudes of Westerners and Africans and that have had a deleterious impact on foreign relations. As a "classic" instance of Europeans blaming Africans for AIDS, the Panos Dossier (1989:76) cited a sensational article in the British *Sunday Telegraph* (September 21, 1986), which claimed that British diplomats in Tanzania, Uganda, and Zambia had warned that African visitors to Britain could be a primary source of infection and should be subjected to blood screening. Despite the British government's disavowal of any plans to screen Zambians, the Zambian minister of health threatened reciprocation and labeled AIDS a capitalist disease. One damaging result of the exchange was that British physicians and researchers working with Zambian colleagues on AIDS projects were told that the collaboration could not continue. The rash of accusations spread to other African countries and led both to denials of the seriousness of the epidemic and to delays in launching control programs. Nigeria tried to wish it away, as the Nigerian magazine *Newswatch* admitted in March 1987, and thus lost precious time in responding to the crisis.

Aside from seeing the attempts to blame them for the epidemic as a political insult, the African governments have had an economic motivation. African ministers in charge of tourism have been worried about the potentially deleterious effect on tourism, a major source of foreign revenue. Zambians attributed the decline of tourist revenues in 1985 to unfavorable reports in the British press concerning the prevalence of AIDS among Zambian students in Britain. The Kenyan government was particularly upset by erroneous media reports originating in Boston, London, and Stockholm concerning the prevalence of AIDS in Kenya. It expressed its anger at the Western press by confiscating copies of the *International Herald Tribune* that carried a *New York Times* story on AIDS in Kenya (Waite 1989).

The Africans' outraged response to what they perceived as racial stereo-typing is eloquently summarized in an article entitled "The Spread of Racism" in the journal *West Africa* (Chirimuuta et al. 1988). The article maintained that the uncontrolled sexuality of black people is a continuing theme of racist mythology used, for example, to justify the lynching of innocent black people in the southern United States. When AIDS first appeared in black people, in the minds of white people it changed almost overnight from a "gay plague" to being an imported Haitian disease and then to being an African disease. Many black people, the authors assert, view the Haitian and African connections with a profound skepticism.

The "blame the foreigner" syndrome found a different expression in the Soviet disinformation campaign (launched in 1985 at the height of the Cold War) directed against the United States. As Nelkin and Gilman (1988:361) report, the AIDS virus was described in articles published in the *Literaturnaya Gazeta*, the official journal of the Soviet Writers Union, as the product of bio-logical warfare scientists at Fort Detrick, Maryland. *Glasnost* brought a reversal of this propaganda tactic in late 1986 and an admission that the USSR also had cases of AIDS. Nelkin and Gilman emphasize that "blaming has always been a means to make mysterious and devastating diseases comprehensible and therefore possibly controllable" and that "perplexing medical questions have always generated hostility." Blaming becomes a political act, and many political leaders confuse medical goals with their ideological assumptions. Thus, exclusionary policies in the form of requiring testing for AIDS antibod-ies are directed at outsiders—in particular, at "immigrants, refugees, aliens, and even foreign students."

A variant of the cross-cultural implications of reactions to the AIDS pan-demic is the ongoing controversy concerning the origins of the virus causing the disease. A particular source of resentment by Africans have been two the-ories, espoused by scientists writing in British scientific journals such as *The Lancet* and the *British Medical Journal*, summarized in American journals such as *Science* and *Scientific American*, and reiterated in press reports. The first the-ory is that AIDS has been endemic to Africa for a long time, perhaps for decades, but was unrecognized until the clustering of cases in recent years. The second is that HIV evolved from a virus found in African green monkeys and was somehow passed on to Africans and thence to the rest of the world. Both theories have been denounced as a residue of a colonialist mentality that sees Africa as both primitive and inferior. The African press generally rejected these theories and espoused the opposite view that AIDS had spread from Europe to Africa. Again, the article quoted above from *West Africa* excoriates the thesis that cases of AIDS in patients from Central Africa who are residing in Europe are proof that AIDS originated in Africa. Although many of these patients had been residing in Europe for a long time, the authors point out, the possibility that "they may have contracted the disease in Europe was not considered." The article concludes with this indictment:

> We would like to believe that the uncritical acceptance of the African connec-
> tion was a simple error of judgement but it seems far more likely that the AIDS
> researchers, the medical experts, the media and the public at large are affected
> by the insidious and frequently unrecognized disease of racism (Chirimuuta et
> al. 1988:312).

One episode in this acrimonious debate is worth noting because of the light it sheds on cultural misperceptions and sensitivities. In an exchange of letters appearing in the *Scientific American*, Muniini Mulera (1989), a Uganda-trained physician, denounced an article in the October 1988 issue, co-authored by Robert C. Gallo and Luc Montagnier. Gallo, of the National Cancer Institute in Bethesda, Maryland, and Montagnier, of the Pasteur Institute, Paris, had reiterated the premise that AIDS had been present in Central Africa for many years. Accusing the authors of ignorance of the demography and history of Central Africa, Mulera pointed out that the migration between city and countryside had been going on at least since the Second World War, that health services in Uganda were "excellent" from 1950 to the end of the 1970s, and that no cases of AIDS had been diagnosed before 1982. Citing a blood-sampling survey carried out between 1976 and 1984 which he believes repudiated the thesis that AIDS originated in Africa, he concluded that we do not know the origin of HIV, "but perpetuating a myth does not help science and only reinforces the ever-present racism and bigotry toward Africans." Gallo and Montagnier replied that they had postulated that (1) the AIDS epidemic had begun in the United States, Haiti, and Central Africa at approximately the same time; (2) HIV has been present in humans for more than 100 years; (3) demographic changes may have spread the disease from smaller, closed groups to larger ones, creating new patterns of the disease; (4) cases were identified in retrospect in Central Africa as early as the 1960s; (5) high rates of infection were found among prostitutes in Rwanda in 1983; (6) retroviruses related to the human AIDS retroviruses were found in African monkeys but never in New World or Asian primates; and (7) the question of the origin of the AIDS virus is obviously related to but different from the factors that govern the epidemic in each region or area. The authors concluded:

> We do not suggest that the virus was transmitted en masse from central Africa to
> other areas or that the people of that region are any more responsible for the
> disease's transmission than, say, the residents of Connecticut are responsible for
> Lyme disease, which in fact was first described in Lyme, Conn. What we postu-
> late as the trigger of the epidemic in central Africa—changing demography and
> behavior—is equally applicable to groups in Europe and the Americas. Histori-
> cally we note that many microbes appear to have originated in Europe and the
> Americas or were first found in humans there.
>   We deeply regret, and in fact do not understand, an interpretation of our
> work and opinions on the origin of HIV that finds bigotry or suggests we blame

anyone, much less an entire continent. In our opinion, HIV–1 very likely originated in a small region of central Africa and HIV–2 in western Africa. This point
is not based on prejudice, nor is it purely academic; it has major long-term medical importance, and we believe it is time to discuss facts openly and honestly
(Gallo & Montagnier 1989:11).

THE POSITIVE RESPONSE: THE GLOBAL
MOBILIZATION AGAINST AIDS

Although the United Nations was slow to mobilize in the wake of the global
threat of AIDS, in the first decade of the pandemic the UN system mounted
what it described in its literature as one of the few genuinely international
efforts in human history. Given the brief history of the pandemic, this development was characterized as extraordinary by Jonathan Mann (1988b). He
identified three significant periods in the evolution of a global attack on
AIDS.

The first, starting in the mid–1970s, was the time of the silent pandemic,
during which the HIV infection spread—undetected, unrecognized—
through five continents.

The second was a time of discovery, occurring, fortunately, at a time
when scientific knowledge had developed the tools to detect human
pathogens of the type that ultimately was identified as causing AIDS. The
description of the AIDS syndrome in 1981 initiated another period of discovery during which the modes in which the disease was transmitted were
defined, the specific causative virus was discovered, and the ability to identify
antiviral antibodies was developed. In turn, the presence of antibodies to the
HIV infection revealed that large numbers of individuals were infected—
although asymptomatically—and that there was a long latency period between
infection and the appearance of symptoms of the full-fledged disease. This
new information was brought together and made public at the first international conference in 1985. Its effect, according to Mann, was to mark a dawn-
ing awareness of the broad impact of AIDS and to stir feelings of a powerful
international solidarity.

The third period has been characterized by a global mobilization of scientific and public health resources against the pandemic through the establishment in February 1987 of a Special Programme on AIDS, under the leadership of WHO, later to be renamed the Global Programme on AIDS (GPA).

The establishment of the program marked a turning point, as the Panos
Dossier (1989:92–93) notes: "From this point on, the climate of world opinion
on AIDS seemed to change almost overnight." Until then, national sensibili-
ties prevailed; some countries would not acknowledge publicly that they were
affected, for the reasons discussed above. Indeed, this continued to be the
case throughout 1987, but "the tide had turned." The problem faced by WHO
was to launch a massive effort on a global scale for which there had been few

precedents. The campaign against smallpox, which was launched in 1967 and which is considered to have achieved its eradication in 1980, is such a precedent. The smallpox campaign cost $81 million. Obviously, the worldwide cost of the war on AIDS, impossible to calculate at this early stage, will be enormously greater.[3]

THE WORLD HEALTH ORGANIZATION GLOBAL PROGRAMME ON AIDS

The principal role of the GPA is to coordinate national efforts at surveillance, prevention, and research, and to function as a resource for governments in their efforts to develop national control plans. Its three major avowed goals are (1) to halt the spread of the pandemic by preventing new HIV infections; (2) to provide support for individuals already infected; and (3) to unite national and international efforts to stem the tide of AIDS. The GPA coordinates worldwide surveillance; reports are received from WHO collaborating centers throughout the world as well as from individual ministries of health. By 1990, a total of 181 countries were reporting AIDS cases to what is, in effect, a global data bank.

The GPA developed into a fairly large organization, with sections devoted to program support, surveillance, health education, social and behavioral research. biomedical research, and epidemiological research (World Health Organization 1988). Coordinated by the GPA, both industrialized and developing countries have launched ambitious and aggressive prevention and control programs. The specific objectives of these efforts have been (1) to prevent sexual transmission of AIDS; (2) to screen blood and blood products; (3) to improve the sterilization of skin-piercing instruments; (4) to improve the management of HIV infection; and (5) to strengthen the monitoring and examination of data on AIDS. In implementing these activities, the GPA has facilitated, encouraged, or co-sponsored a number of regional conferences in Africa, the Americas, Southeast Asia, Europe, the eastern Mediterranean region, and the western Pacific, providing a mechanism for the exchange of expertise, field experience, and ideas for health professionals.

One signal accomplishment of the GPA, according to the Africanists Barnett and Blaikie (1992:17), has been the establishment of an AIDS database on both mortality and infection which—even if it is flawed—serves as a basis for developing national reporting systems and national AIDS policies.

One of the GPA's vital functions since its inception has been to alert the World Bank concerning the latest assessments of the future course of the pandemic. Under the leadership of Jonathan Mann, its first director, the organization became a catalyst for informing the world concerning the dangers of the pandemic and for launching programs to contain it. Mann championed a nontraditional public health approach to AIDS which transcended immediate concerns with the health aspects of the pandemic and which stressed the centrality of human rights in all its strategies. The distinguishing feature of the first phase of the GPA program has been a concern not only for the toll in human suffering and death but also for the social burden of stigma and the resulting discrimination against AIDS victims. The strategy of combating the disease itself went beyond distributing condoms to emphasizing a broader behavioral and social science approach, which included steering the GPA toward supporting nongovernmental organizations (NGOs) throughout the world.

In March 1990, Mann resigned from his position as director of the GPA, citing philosophical differences with his superior, Hiroshi Nakajima, the director general of WHO, who had cut the GPA budget—thus putting it on a more equal footing with other WHO programs. Under the leadership of Mann's successor, Michael Merson, also a public health physician, the GPA has changed in both style and direction. The style is more managerial, which some observers consider appropriate for consolidating and sustaining the GPA programs within the WHO bureaucracy. A more fundamental difference is a change in philosophy. Merson's objective is to warn those developing countries where the HIV virus has not yet established a bridgehead. He argues that if these vulnerable countries wait for AIDS cases to appear, "it is too darn late." He stresses a policy of encouraging condom use, developing targeted educational programs, and paying increased attention to the treatment of all sexually transmitted diseases. Under his administration, less attention is paid to the behavioral aspects of AIDS; funds for behavioral research have accordingly been reduced.

Mann takes issue with this narrower focus, arguing against the temptation to define away the pandemic by calling it a central problem of the industrialized world but just another endemic problem of the developing world. He argues against blaming those whose behavior is not changing rapidly enough, and he asserts that to wait "for technology to rescue us from ourselves" is tantamount to letting the pandemic dominate us (*Science*, News and Comment, October 25, 1991:512). The reality of the second phase of the GPA's stewardship is that in the second decade of the pandemic it faces the battle against AIDS with a reduced staff and reduced funds at a time when a concern with the international aspects no longer is front page news throughout the world.[4]

THE ANNUAL AIDS CONFERENCES: AN INTERNATIONAL FORUM

WHO provides the leadership for creating a unique international forum through annual conferences on AIDS which are cosponsored by the WHO and host countries. It was through these conferences that the dimensions of the pandemic—its commonalties and diverse features—and its scientific, medical, social, economic, and cultural implications emerged. Each has attracted increasingly larger numbers of participants—epidemiologists, virologists, public health specialists, physicians, statisticians, and field workers in nongovernmental organizations—from around the world. Increasingly, the conferences have included social scientists, especially behavioral psychologists, demographers, economists, political scientists, and sociologists. And there is always a large international press corps in attendance.

The first international conference on AIDS was held in Atlanta, Georgia, in 1985. It was concerned primarily with scientific topics (molecular biology, virology, immunology, epidemiology, clinical medicine, and public health) and drew some 2,000 participants. It was at the second conference in Paris, in 1986, that news from the developing world revealed that AIDS was indeed an international problem without an immediate solution, requiring a global response. Realizing that progress toward developing vaccines for immunization as well as drugs for treatment would not take place in the immediate future, the conference planners began to stress the social aspects of AIDS.

The third conference in Washington in 1987 took on political overtones. President Reagan, bowing to public pressure, delivered a speech on AIDS the evening before the conference, and Vice President Bush addressed the opening ceremony. Gay activist groups began to draw attention to the human impact of the disease through demonstrations outside the conference hall.

At the fourth conference, held in Stockholm in 1988 and attended by over 7,000 people, the program not only stressed humanitarian concerns for the victims of the disease but also identified emerging social, ethical, and legal implications.

At the fifth conference, held in Montreal in 1989 and attended by 11,000 people, conflict between activist groups—agitating for more rapid U.S. government action in research and treatment and the conference organizers became quite apparent. The sessions of the conference named "AIDS, Society, and Behaviour" reflected these social concerns. Individual panels discussed the impact of AIDS on the individual and on families, the ethics of testing for HIV, the role of religion and the media, the problems of AIDS in the workplace, the impact of AIDS on minorities, and patients' rights to privacy—among a host of topics demonstrating the social implications of the pandemic.

The need to respond to the changing nature of the concern for AIDS was echoed by Alastair Clayton (1989), director general of the Canadian Federal Centre for AIDS, as the Montreal conference began. Noting that some 70 percent of the abstracts submitted were biomedical, he said he would like the ratio to be 50–50. The signal distinguishing characteristic of each successive conference, however, has been the inclusion and increasing recognition of the roles of PWAs (persons with AIDS) and organized gay activist groups. Robert Wachtler (1991), a physician AIDS specialist who was one of the principal organizers of the 1990 San Francisco conference, refers to the preceding

Montreal conference as a landmark of the activist movement. It was at Montreal, he observes, that the activists "exploded." In planning the next conference in San Francisco, he reports, the increasingly formidable presence of these activist groups in the newly created field of AIDS politics was a dominant concern.

The 1990 San Francisco conference may have represented the peak of the emphasis on community and policy issues, but the focal issue that emerged during the months of planning that preceded it was an international one. Wachtler describes how the barring of a Dutch delegate to the conference under the U.S. immigration rule prohibiting seropositives from entering the country became a rallying point for opposition to the law.

Opposition to the ban on seropositives became the focus of international criticism of the U.S. policy. On November 23, 1989, the International Red Cross announced its intention to boycott the San Francisco conference. Despite a subsequent waiver in visa procedures that permitted seropositive travelers to attend the conference if they admitted being infected and accepted having their passport stamped with this information, the boycott was joined by the International AIDS Society, the World Hemophilia Association, the governments of France and Switzerland, and ultimately the European Community. As Wachtler reports, the discriminatory travel policy offered Europeans, and especially the French, the opportunity to "wrap themselves in the flag of righteousness and elevate the travel restriction issue to a test of moral integrity." The U.S. national organization of PWAs also joined the boycott.[5] In response, the Department of Health and Human Services and the Immigration and Naturalization Service amended the wording of the travel restriction to avoid documentation of the applicant's status and thus to protect the confidentiality of this information.

Yielding to further international and domestic pressures, the Department of Justice[6] issued a travel plan exempting individuals who applied for a ten-day stay to attend the conference from revealing their HIV status—"in the public interest." This compromise effectively lifted the boycott of attendance at the San Francisco conference.

The seventh AIDS conference was held in Florence, Italy, in 1991. Observers at the conference, which had 8,000 participants, noted a sea change in the tone of the event. The conference was primarily scientific in nature, showing a reduced emphasis on sessions devoted to social policy issues and an increased sense of failure at efforts in education and behavior change (*New York Times*, June 17, 1991:7). The Bush administration's decision to finance the travel of only half the number of scientists originally scheduled to attend was criticized by attending scientists from all over the world.[7] The Italian chairman of the conference stressed that the exchange of ideas among scientists was a crucial aspect of the meeting and he noted that the participants would sorely miss the opportunities for discussions with the absent American scientists.

Some participants at the Florence conference launched sharp attacks on the U.S. government's continuing policy of restricting the entry of infected travelers. Organizers of the next conference, which was scheduled to be sponsored by Harvard University and convened in Boston in 1992, warned that they would cancel the conference, in response to the mounting criticism, if the restrictions were not removed.[8] The European Community again expressed its concern over the restrictions. But an undercurrent of questioning by an increasing number of scientists concerning the costs and value of the conferences was also evident. In fact, in recent years more scientists have chosen to release their research findings to professional journals rather than in presentations at these conferences. However, Anthony Fauci of the U.S. National Institute of Allergy and Infectious Disease, the ranking U.S. government scientist at the Florence conference, voiced disappointment that more U.S. scientists had not been able to attend and noted that some scientists had funded their own travel (*New York Times*, June 17, 1991:7).

At the conference, Jonathan Mann voiced the criticism that the international AIDS program was being affected by complacency and foot dragging and he called for a renewal of the international response. He also criticized the lack of papers on the social impact of AIDS. According to Oliver Morton, the science editor of *The Economist*, "in Florence, the sense of urgency that was common to all the previous conferences seems to have faded. It is not gone. . . . But it is not the progressive force it once was" (quoted in *AIDS & Society*, July/August 1991:2).

In August 1991, the Harvard AIDS Institute, the organizers of the planned 1992 Boston conference, announced that because of the travel restrictions it was canceling the conference. In September, it was announced that the conference would be held in Amsterdam: the Netherlands had no HIV–related restrictions on travel or immigration (*Science*, Briefings, September 27, 1991:1484). In the official announcement, the Harvard-Amsterdam organizers stated that the goal of the conference would be to present new results of basic, clinical, and epidemiological research and to help strengthen understanding of the social dimensions of the epidemic.

The Amsterdam AIDS conference, held July 19–22, 1992, was the largest thus far; it was attended by some 12,000 individuals.[9] It was also expensive, costing $25 million according to some reports. The day before it opened, an editorial in *The Lancet*, deploring this expense, declared that "the era of megaconferences [on AIDS] should now end" ("AIDS: An Opportunity Not to Be Lost" 1992:148).

The highlights of the Amsterdam conference were public policy issues: human rights, women and AIDS, the role of nongovernmental organizations (NGOs) in the developing world's struggle against AIDS, and the emerging roles of organizations of persons with AIDS (PWAs)—issues that had largely been left hanging in Montreal. For the first time, women's issues received focused attention. The inclusion of activists in the program made protests less disruptive than in the past: Most of the protests were aimed at the shortcomings of the U.S. government's leadership in HIV–AIDS issues. The discovery of a possible "new virus" dominated the scientific sessions and captured the attention of the international press.

Press reports of the conference referred to a pervading feeling of pessimism concerning the future—a pessimism that had first become manifest at the Florence conference. As Lawrence K. Altman, the physician-reporter of the *New York Times* noted, the conference ended on a somber note, generated by the growing recognition that "AIDS is yielding its secrets slowly and . . . the full dimensions of the puzzle are not known" (*New York Times,* July 26, 1992:1).

Critics of the Amsterdam conference stressed the fact that 85 percent of the participants came from the industrialized countries. In the words of one observer, the conference was "the regional meeting of the North" (Berkley 1992:3).

A more trenchant and radical criticism was voiced by the Australian Dennis Altman (1993:7), who, following the Amsterdam conference, complained that the international AIDS conferences "are largely U.S. national conferences, at which the rest of us are often onlookers." American predominance is not confined to scientists and doctors but includes activists as well. "Western and nonwestern community activists do not for the most part share the same priorities," he added. Furthermore, he noted, "the issues around AIDS in the rich world are increasingly driven by the latest developments in medical technology, which is irrelevant to the great majority of those infected in the developing world." In order for the developing world to be heard at these conferences, Altman believes, national quotas will have to be imposed to prevent the domination of any one country's agenda.

The ninth international conference on AIDS was held in Berlin, June 7–11, 1993, and drew 14,000 participants. This conference also sounded an alarm concerning the unchecked spread of the AIDS virus throughout the world. Again, the dominant note was pessimism concerning the rate of scientific progress in dealing with HIV infection and AIDS disease. Lawrence Altman, in summarizing the conference for the *New York Times* (June 12, 1993:5), quoted Michael Merson as saying that "we must accept that our scientific advances today are coming in small steps, not in leaps and bounds."

Scientists working on the development of a vaccine reported new obstacles. The AIDS virus is everchanging: five, perhaps six major genetic subtypes of the main virus (HIV–1) have been identified. Moreover, different subtypes of HIV predominate in different parts of the world, only to be replaced by other, mutating strains that become dominant. This phenomenon has already been observed in Thailand and in South America. The Swedish epidemiologist Lars O. Kallings raised the possibility that in developing a vaccine, scientists may need to monitor HIV as they now do the influenza virus, adjusting the vaccine periodically to target the latest mutations.

News presented at the meeting about the effectiveness of anti–HIV drugs was also disheartening. A large-scale European study whose results questioned the value of using AZT to delay the onset of AIDS symptoms in HIV–infected people had been made public a month before the conference and had been criticized by American physicians. At the conference, additional data on the design of the study satisfied many critics.

Summarizing the conference, Altman wrote that only "an eternal optimist" would have left the meetings believing that new drugs would be available in time to save the lives of the 14 million people now infected throughout the world or that a vaccine would be developed in time to prevent the infection of the more than 30 million people predicted by the year 2000 (*New York Times,* June 15, 1993:C-1). The one clear note sounded at Berlin is that the only hope of stemming the pandemic at this time is through prevention.

The international AIDS conferences have come under attack from critics who claim they are counterproductive because of their huge size and circus-like atmosphere. On the eve of the Berlin conference, the British journal *Nature* called for their end, as *The Lancet* had done a year earlier before the Amsterdam conference. Kallings, however, speaking in Berlin, defended the conferences, maintaining that they serve a vital function because of the degree of involvement of both persons with AIDS (PWAs) and scientists—a feature that distinguishes them from other conferences that exclude patients from their conceptualization and planning. The question, Kallings said, is whether the next meeting in Yokohama in 1994 will report examples of how policies for preventing the spread of the epidemic have been changed and proof that these efforts have reduced high-risk behavior. . . .

A RATIONALE FOR INTERNATIONAL COLLABORATION

Nicholas A. Christakis (1990:329), a public health physician, identifies the common interests and divergent needs that mandate an international response. "Unlike other so-called international health problems, such as malaria and smallpox," he points out, "AIDS strikes the developing and developed world with equal vengeance and forces all nations to consider their common interests in the solution of international health problems." The AIDS pandemic, he notes, "provides a new opportunity to view health as an international phenomenon, one that is best addressed by policies with international dimensions" (329).

In identifying AIDS as an international health problem, Christakis raises the following questions: Which aspects of the spread of the disease need international attention? What should the national and international objectives of AIDS control be? Why should the international impact of AIDS concern single nations? Why, for example, should the United States be interested in devoting efforts to control AIDS elsewhere rather than in concentrating solely on its own epidemic? One answer to these questions is that AIDS is a pandemic, and a pandemic disease cannot be addressed in the same manner as an epidemic disease. AIDS transcends national boundaries in the sense that it occurs worldwide. Yet the fact of worldwide occurrence in itself does not make it an international problem:

> There a distinction between a *worldwide* problem and an *international* problem. The latter has an important feature in addition to worldwide occurrence. This feature is the direct interrelatedness of the problem in one country with the problem in another or of the cause of the problem in one country with the effect in another (Christakis 1990:330).

In this sense AIDS is typical of other international problems such as pollution, ozone depletion, arms proliferation, and hunger. All of these require international approaches. By the same token, "narrow, nationalistic" policies directed at controlling the spread of AIDS are not effective.

A host of factors arising out of the increasing interdependence of the modern world are contributing to the spread of AIDS and make an international approach to control essential. Among these are the immigration and travel of HIV–infected individuals, trade in defective condoms and antibody testing kits, international transport of consequences of AIDS, as much as the causes of AIDS, have both common origins and divergent manifestations and require international collaboration in sharing experience, insights, and approaches to solutions.

A number of aspects of the AIDS pandemic are crucial to its understanding. First is the special trauma resulting from AIDS attacks against specific subgroups in societies throughout the world—young adults, the disadvantaged, ethnic minorities, and the children who are victims of congenital AIDS and whose drug-addicted mothers are equally doomed. Second is the strain imposed on health services that deal with these groups—in rich countries like the United States as well as in the economically deprived developing countries. Third are the ubiquitous expressions of prejudice and the practice of discrimination in the workplace against individuals suspected of being carriers. Fourth, we must consider a host of issues that have surfaced since AIDS began to exact its human toll: for example, devising control measures in penal situations, in the military, in public schools. Finally, certain ethical issues are becoming manifest as a result of the clash between individual rights to privacy and the interest of society in protecting itself against the spread of the disease.

Speaking from the standpoint of a sociologist, Richard Rockwell (1988:5223) articulated a further rationale for examining the social implications of AIDS. "Even if no one else is ever again infected," he maintained, "the pandemic will have historically significant consequences. The lethal virus does not have to kill in hundreds of millions before we see social impacts beyond the lives it takes, and the social and economic burden their illnesses and deaths impose."

NOTES

1. For additional details of this controversy, see the later section of this chapter, "The annual AIDS conferences: An international forum."

2. Ergas called attention to another potentially inhibiting effect on international relations of foreign suspicions of Americans as transmitters of AIDS, that is, the U.S. Department of State announcement in December 1986 that a test for HIV seropositivity would be required of all employees and their dependents stationed overseas.

3. For further details of the Global Programme on AIDS, see Chapter 8 of the Panos Dossier (1989).

4. According to Earickson (1990), the growing pandemic coincides with a period of decreasing Western support for WHO and of decreasing U.S. support for its sister agency the Pan American Health Organization. The United States has thus far made only what has been called a modest contribution of funds to WHO earmarked for the AIDS program.

5. On December 12, 1989, June Osborn, as chair of the U.S. National Commission on AIDS, labeled the restrictions "counterproductive, discriminatory, and a waste of resources. . . . They reinforce the false impression that AIDS and HIV infection are a general threat when in fact they are sharply restricted in their mode of transmission" (quoted in Wachtler 1991:119).

6. The Immigration and Naturalization Service is a component of the Department of Justice.

7. The U.S. government supported the attendance of more than 700 scientists at the San Francisco conference. It reduced that number to 400 for the Florence meeting because of travel costs. New budget restrictions imposed by the Congress subsequently forced the Public Health Service to cut the 400 figure in half.

8. Commenting on the continuing AIDS ban, an editorial in the *New York Times* (June 19, 1991:A24) stated that it is a "travesty that the United States, with one of the largest AIDS–infected populations in the world, has taken a stance that implies the danger comes from abroad."

9. The eighth international conference on AIDS was held in conjunction with the STD World Congress and was sponsored by Harvard University and the Dutch AIDS Foundation: co-sponsors were the International AIDS Society and WHO.

REFERENCES

Altman, Dennis. 1993. Conference Opinion: Amsterdam. *AIDS & Society* (January/February):7.

Barnett, Tony, and Piers Blaikie. 1992. *AIDS in Africa: Its Present and Future Impact*. New York: Guilford Press.

Berkley, Seth. 1992. Amsterdam Viewpoint: Costly Regional AIDS Conference for the North. *AIDS & Society* (July/August):3–4.

Christakis, Nicholas A. 1990. "Responding to a Pandemic: International Interests in AIDS Control." In *Living with AIDS*, edited by Stephen R. Graubard. Cambridge, Mass.: MIT Press.

Clayton, Alastair J. 1989. "Building a New Perspective on AIDS." Interview in *AIDS '89 Bulletin*. Fifth International Conference on AIDS, Montreal, June 4–9.

Chirimuuta, Richard, et al. 1988. "The Spread of Racism." In *The AIDS Reader*, edited by Loren K. Clarke and Malcolm Potts. Boston: Brandon Publishing Co.

Ergas, Yasmine. 1987. The Social Consequences of the AIDS Epidemic. Social Science Research Council, *Items* 41 (December):33–39.

Gallo, Robert C., and Luc Montagnier. 1988. The Authors Respond. *Scientific American* 260 (June):10–11.

Krisber, Paul, and Harry Blaney. 1987. AIDS International: Disease Is Altering the Nation's Foreign Policy. *The Bergen (N.J.) Record*. (October 16). [Reprinted from the *Washington Post*.]

Mann, Jonathan. 1988b. "The Global Picture of AIDS." Unpublished paper delivered at the Fourth International Conference on AIDS, Stockholm. June 12–16.

Misztal, Barbara, and David Moss, eds. 1990. *Action on AIDS: National Policies in Comparative Perspective*. Westport, Conn.:

Mulera, Muniini. 1989. Letter to the Editors. *Scientific American* 26 (June):10.

Nelkin, Dorothy, and Sander L. Gilman. 1988. Placing Blame for Devastating Disease. *Social Research* 55 (3):361–378.

Panos Dossier. 1989. *AIDS and the Third World*. Published in association with the Norwegian Red Cross by the Panos Institute. Philadelphia: New Society Publishers.

Rockwell, Richard C. 1988. Social Impacts of the HIV Epidemic. *AIDS* 2 (Supplement 1):S223–S227.

Tomasevski, Katarina. 1992. "AIDS and Human Rights." In *AIDS in the World*, edited by Jonathan Mann et al., 538–573. Cambridge, Mass.: Harvard Univ. Press.

Wachtler, Robert M. 1991. *The Fragile Coalition: Scientists, Activists, and AIDS*. New York: St. Martin's Press.

Waite, Gloria. 1988. "The Politics of Disease," In *AIDS in Africa*, edited by Norman N. Miller and Richard C. Rockwell. Lewiston, Me.: Edwin Mellen Press.